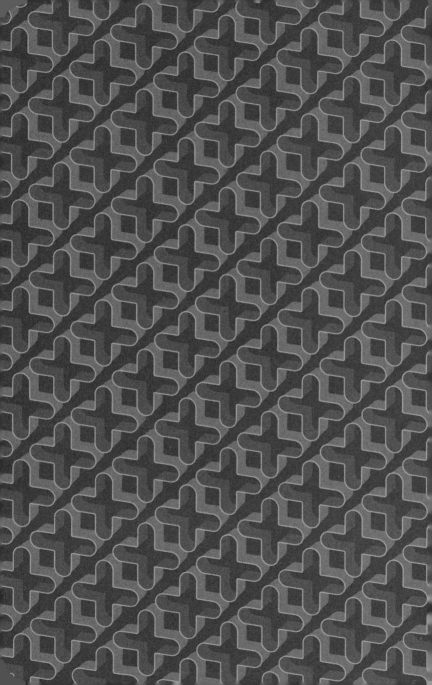

ADVANCE PRAISE

"There is no health without mental health, so it's refreshing that *Positive Mental Health* takes a whole person, holistic approach to the topic through the multiple lenses of physical, mental and financial health and wellbeing."

Louise Aston, Wellbeing Director,
Business in the Community

"The link between physical and mental wellbeing has always existed, but in today's society the recognition has never been stronger and there is a huge amount of scientific research to prove it as well. Though the relationship between the two is complex, there is no denying that exercise can brighten your mood, increase endorphins, reduce stress and even heighten self-esteem. Some doctors are even now prescribing exercise as a means to treat stress, anxiety and depression. Given that most of our time is spent in a working environment it is now more important than ever for corporate organizations to encourage physical activity. A healthier and happier workplace is, of course, a win-win for everyone."

Pietro Carmignani, CEO in UK & IE, Gympass

"It is widely accepted that physical health has a strong correlation with positive mental health; key aspects such as mood, self-esteem and anxiety reduction are areas that benefit from exercise and activity. Books like *Positive Mental Health* discuss these important areas, and many more, and so contribute to the health and wellbeing debates in a very constructive way – increasing awareness and decreasing the stigma associated with mental ill health has to be a good thing, right?"

Dan Moore, Managing Director, Moore Fitness

"This book is, without doubt, a great way of supporting individuals who want to have a toolkit to improve their mental health – I'm delighted to recommend it."

Eugene Farrell, Chair, UK Employee Assistance Professionals Association

Published by
LID Publishing Limited
The Record Hall, Studio 204,
16-16a Baldwins Gardens,
London EC1N 7RJ, UK

info@lidpublishing.com
www.lidpublishing.com

A member of:

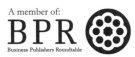

www.businesspublishersroundtable.com

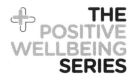

© Dr Shaun Davis & Andrew Kinder, 2019
© LID Publishing Limited, 2019

Printed in the Czech Republic by Finidr

ISBN: 978-1-912555-55-0

Cover and page design: Caroline Li

POSITIVE MENTAL HEALTH

OVERCOMING MENTAL HEALTH PROBLEMS

DR SHAUN DAVIS
& ANDREW KINDER

MADRID | MEXICO CITY | LONDON
NEW YORK | BUENOS AIRES
BOGOTA | SHANGHAI | NEW DELHI

Develop a better quality of life, both physically and mentally with...

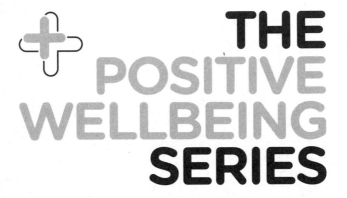

THE
POSITIVE
WELLBEING
SERIES

FOR OTHER TITLES IN THE SERIES:

+ Resilience
+ Stress management
+ Health
+ Physical energy
+ Mental energy
+ Emotional energy

+ Nutrition
+ Fulfilling aspirations
+ Self awareness
+ Strengths training/
  wellness in the workplace

thepositivewellbeingseries.com

CONTENTS

ACKNOWLEDGMENTS

We would like to acknowledge Liz Guilford and the whole LID production team who have contributed to making this book a success. Shaun would like to dedicate the book to Greig for his continuing support in all he does, to Dan his personal trainer who helps him 'walk the talk' and to all the fantastic employees of Royal Mail Group. Andrew dedicates the book to Jane and his family for their great support over many years and to his many clients who have made their own journeys to improved mental health.

FOREWORD

The concept of sustaining positive mental health is something that is testing societies and businesses worldwide today and the challenge of tackling the many evolving pressures within our modern lives is something that we each have a responsibility to support.

If I think about the different pressures faced by my two teenage daughters compared with those I faced at their age, it is a stark reminder of how demanding transitions can be during our lives – from starting our first job, to relationships and family, to changing career, to handling bereavement, to moving house and everything in between – and with so much of this being tracked by social media, the need for resilience and good mental health has never been more apparent to me.

Fundamentally, good mental health is relevant to all of us – for ourselves, within our families, for friends, colleagues or employees – and without doubt, having good mental health is critical in terms of enjoying and thriving at work. It is also a growing necessity for organizations to engage and take active and proactive steps to promote good mental health and resilience on a day-to-day basis, regardless of gender, sexual orientation, religion, age or any other factor.

I am encouraged that, in recent years, the subject of mental health has grown in visibility. We are now able to speak openly about mental health issues in order to get the right support and it seems that the message is getting through. With instances of poor mental health being reported more frequently we're increasingly prepared to raise and report mental health issues, which is actually a huge step forward.

Poor mental health has become the greatest cause of workplace absence and more organizations are adopting a proactive stance to support good mental health, as well as ensuring rehabilitation is in place both inside and outside the workplace through a variety of wellbeing initiatives and incentives. This should be applauded and expanded and it makes economic sense: the concept that a 'happy employee is a productive employee' also proves the business rationale for this new focus.

Perhaps some of the most important relationships we have at work are with our line manager and close colleagues. Where organizations are able to successfully promote and support good mental health at this 'local' level for each of us, it's possible that they can fundamentally change the landscape of mental health, developing understanding and practical skills to create the resilience that is necessary for us all to cope with the demands of the world today. We each need to play our part in understanding and supporting each other on a day-to-day basis and, as part of this, I am hugely proud of the work we do at Optima Health to support our people and clients in the arena of mental health from proactive mental wellbeing initiatives, through Employee Assistance Programmes to counselling and specialist services, such as EMDR and (e)CBT.

This book is a great guide to understanding more about handling the pressures of life and supporting those who are experiencing demanding transitions and mental health challenges. It provides a practical outlook and gives tools that can be used to support ourselves as individuals, as well as those we work alongside and our families and friends.

I wish you personally all the best as you consider this most important societal challenge and what it means for you and those around you, as well as the positive impact you can make for yourself and others.

Simon Arnold
Chief Executive Officer
Optima Health

INTRODUCTION

We have written our new book, *Positive Mental Health: Overcoming Mental Health Problems* to highlight the challenges that many of us face when it comes to mental health, regardless of our gender, age, sexual or gender orientation and the demographic that we live in. Our aim is to help readers to identify how they can improve, nurture and protect their mental health.

But, importantly, it has also been written with a conversation in mind; perhaps you have been looking for help from those at work or at home. Or perhaps you could start a conversation with someone who needs support. Asking someone how they really are can unlock a helpful and life-changing discussion about mental health. Through this book, we hope we can facilitate this.

Too often we take our mental health for granted. Each of us is somewhere on the mental health spectrum and taking care of our psychological and emotional wellbeing is the equivalent of looking after our physical health by good nutrition, quality sleep and staying as active as we can be.

This book is a call to action with chapters on taking charge of your mental health and understanding some specific mental health issues such as stress, trauma, anxiety and depression. It also looks at our mental health at specific points of our life, including parenthood, the menopause, relationship breakdown and even leaving home for the first time. It also examines our mental health at work, how we can help ourselves and what support we can expect from our colleagues and employer.

You can dip in and out of the topics that are relevant to you. But for the longer term, there are some key factors that you can adopt to maintain your mental health on an ongoing basis:

- **Eat a well-balanced diet:** Make sure that you are eating lots of fresh, unprocessed food and drinking plenty of water. Taking care of yourself physically will pay dividends for your mental wellbeing in the long term.

- **Watch how much you're drinking:** Drinking too much alcohol, as well as taking drugs, puts pressure on your physical health and despite the initial high, will leave you feeling depressed, sluggish and tired later. These drugs may also be addictive and therefore highly corrosive to our wellbeing.

- **Take some exercise:** Get moving with physical exercise at least three times a week to produce those 'feel good' endorphins, and boost your physical health.

- **Find a way to relax:** Whether it's yoga or meditation or making time for breathing exercises, find a way to relax to clear your mind and take a step back from what might be causing you stress.

- **Avoid negativity:** Constant negative thinking stops you from enjoying life. Take actions to learn to think positively, perhaps seeking advice from a professional counsellor or coach, or your doctor.

- **Develop a positive outlook:** If you approach what's in front of you with a positive outlook your approach to challenges will dramatically change and you're likely to see opportunities rather than problems.

- **Make time for yourself and your interests or hobbies:** Taking time out can help to re-charge depleted energy and find resources to cope with other areas of your life.

- **Manage your stress:** You're not likely to ever fully remove stress or anxiety so the next best thing is to learn how to manage and reduce it. If you suspect your stress levels are too high, it's probably the right time to get help.

- **Live in the moment and go with the flow:** Try not to dwell on the past or worry about the future, it'll only increase your stress levels, so focus on appreciating the present and where you are right now.

- **Sleep hygiene:** Not sleeping well negatively impacts decision making, mood and the ability to put things into perspective. Make a difference by analysing how to improve your sleep hygiene.

As a society and a community, there is still a lot to do when it comes to starting a conversation about mental health. But we each have to start somewhere. Take it from us, mental health problems can affect anyone – mental health doesn't discriminate but fortunately there are publications, people and organizations who can and will help you. You have nothing to be ashamed of and together we can make a lasting difference.

Dr Shaun Davis
Global Director of Safety,
Health, Wellbeing
& Sustainability
Royal Mail Group

Andrew Kinder
Professional Head of
Mental Health Services
Optima Health

PART 1

UNDER-STANDING YOUR MENTAL HEALTH

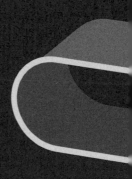

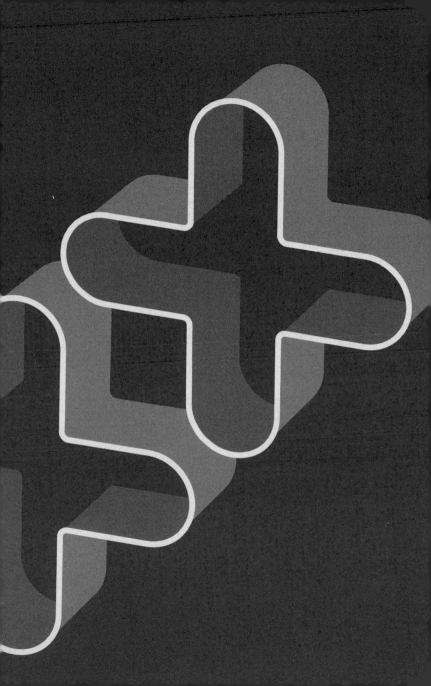

HOW MENTAL HEALTH AFFECTS US

Our mental health encompasses our emotional, psychological and social wellbeing. It affects and influences how we think, feel and act towards ourselves and other people, and shapes how we respond and relate to other people, situations and circumstances. Our mental health is also a key factor that impacts the decisions and choices we make in our lives.

Our mental health is what enables each of us to cope with the 'normal' stresses of our everyday lives.

When mental health is affected by the pressures of life we can develop mental health problems. This can happen to anyone, regardless of age, gender, ethnicity or social group. It's generally accepted that one in four people in the UK experience a mental health problem at some point in their lives. Mental health problems can range from feeling down, and common disorders such as anxiety and depression, to less common but more severe conditions that include bipolar disorder and schizophrenia.

It's really important to understand from the outset that mental health problems can happen to anyone.

Mental health struggles can emerge very suddenly, develop as the result of a specific event or rear their head gradually and worsen over time. Some mental health conditions can be persistent and may be classed as a 'disability' while others might come and go, giving you 'good' and 'bad' days. But with the right support, those diagnosed with mental health conditions can still enjoy a healthy, productive and happy life. In fact, often you can recover completely or learn to manage the symptoms and live a fulfilling life.

Our mental health, just like our physical health, is impacted by a range of factors, environments and experiences. Some of these are likely to be out of our control, whereas others can definitely be influenced by you and those around you.

Some of the most common contributors to mental health issues are biological factors, such as a family history of mental health problems. Other factors might include education, levels of self-awareness and life experiences, such as childhood events, or incidents such as trauma or abuse. These factors can be influenced and ameliorated.

Where you work and what you do for work can also have a negative impact on your mental health. Unmanageable workloads or demands, poorly defined job roles and responsibilities, lack of control over work, an unhealthy work-life balance, poor relationships with your managers or colleagues, organizational change or job insecurity, a lack of variety in work and a lack of career opportunities all potentially contribute to mental ill health. However, it is our view that well-structured and meaningful work can be really good for our mental health and we pick this point up later in the book.

Throughout your lifetime – and sometimes even during the course of a day – it is perfectly normal for your mental health to fluctuate. Sometimes it will be good and other times you might need support, space or a little time to get things back on track. It is also possible that, while your mental health is generally good, you also feel stressed or anxious about something.

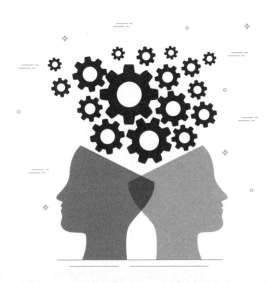

One in four
people in the
UK experience
a mental health
problem at
some point in
their lives.

DO YOU THINK YOU MIGHT HAVE A MENTAL HEALTH PROBLEM?

Mental health is unique to each individual and when we have a mental health problem, the way it presents itself through signs and symptoms are unique too. Despite this, there are several common indicators that could suggest that you have a mental health problem, including:

- Mood swings
- Low mood, feeling numb or sad, or like nothing matters
- Personality change
- Self-harm or suicidal thinking or behaviours
- Reduced concentration, reasoning or decision-making ability
- Difficulty understanding or relating to circumstances or other people
- Detachment from reality; delusional, paranoid feelings or experiencing hallucinations
- Excessive anger, aggression or violent behaviour
- Increased intake of alcohol, tobacco, drugs or medication
- Eating too much or too little
- Withdrawal and isolation; pulling away from people and regular activities

- Lack of interest or motivation
- Tearfulness or feeling sad for no obvious reason
- Irritability
- Excessive tiredness; having little or no energy
- Feeling anxious, on edge, upset, worried or scared
- Being unable to perform daily tasks

Additionally, these symptoms may also indicate that you're going through some form of difficulty or physical illness. It's also important to acknowledge that each specific mental health condition will have its own precise signs and symptoms. That said, considering the broader indicators listed here and recognizing them in yourself or someone close to you is a fantastic starting point to getting some help.

So, if any of these symptoms sound familiar, it is probably time to talk and reach out to a trusted friend, colleague or someone at home, or even a professional who can help you get on the road to recovery.

IDENTIFYING WHAT'S AFFECTING YOUR MENTAL HEALTH

You can't start on the road to recovery and begin to improve, nurture and enhance positive mental health and wellbeing until you've been able to identify the factors that are having an adverse effect on it.

The first positive thing you can do is to try and understand what is impacting your mental health. One way to do this is to keep a daily record that details how you are feeling at certain points in the day, noting anything that's making you feel stressed or unwell.

There are lots of roles that make up our daily lives, whether it's as a parent, employee, friend, manager, relative or volunteer, for example. The following example explains how to keep a daily record of your feelings in a work situation, but the principle is easily adaptable to any of the roles we find ourselves in throughout our day-to-day lives.

At work, for example, are there looming deadlines or regular meetings with clients or colleagues that you can pinpoint as a trigger for you?

Ask yourself these questions to help record how you're feeling:

- Where were you when you started to feel stressed?
- Was there a particular person or group of people involved?
- How did you react to the situation?
- Did you experience negative thoughts and did you challenge them in any way?

By keeping a record of your feelings after certain situations, you can identify patterns of behaviour that will give you the knowledge to take positive action to help yourself.

Alternatively, if you are struggling to identify the specific stressors that are affecting you, you might want to try a different approach, such as making a note of everything you do and how much time you think you spend on each activity, if you think there is something at work that is affecting your mental health.

Try and include everything in your job role, including responding to emails and the regular meetings you attend, as well as favours you do for co-workers.

Look back at your notes ... can you detect anything that might have caused you stress?

Now you have taken that first step to pinpoint the cause of your mental health issues, you are definitely in a better position to do something positive about them.

THE MENTAL HEALTH GENDER GAP

It is a well-known fact that men, when compared with women, are reluctant to admit to health problems and are less likely to seek professional help. Too often, men contact their doctor or mental health support services as a last resort, when things have reached 'crunch point' and have become too tough for them to cope with any longer.

A survey by Opinion Leader for Men's Mental Health Forum found that 46% of men with mental health concerns would be embarrassed or ashamed to take time off work. Some 52% of this group were concerned that their employer would think badly of them if they took time off due to a mental health concern.

A review of the research conducted into men and mental health confirms that men have a tough time getting to grips with their mental health. It's a very real issue.

- At any given time, 12.5% of men are diagnosed with a common mental health condition, such as anxiety, depression, panic disorder or obsessive-compulsive disorder[1]

- At least one in ten of the male workforce in the UK describes themselves as 'significantly stressed' and 34% of those surveyed agreed, or strongly agreed, that they were 'constantly feeling stressed or under pressure' [Men's Health Forum, 2016]

- Only 50% of men feel comfortable discussing mental health issues [Business in the Community, Mental Health at Work Report 2017]

- Researchers found that 28% of men had not sought help for the last mental health problem they experienced, compared with just 19% of women [Mental Health Foundation, 2016]

- Some 34% of men admitted they would be embarrassed or ashamed to take time off work for mental health concerns, compared with 13% who would be self-conscious about doing so for a physical injury [Men's Health Forum, 2016]

- More than three-quarters (76%) of suicides in the UK are by men [Office for National Statistic], with suicide being the biggest cause of death for men under the age of 45 [Department of Health]

The odds really do seem to be stacked against men who find themselves struggling with their mental health.

But why is dealing with mental health issues such a dramatically different experience for men and women? Some argue that these differences are simply out of our hands and that the way men respond to mental health issues is just part of our genetic make-up.

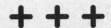

WHILST THIS DEBATE WILL UNDOUBTEDLY CONTINUE, THERE ARE SOME FACTORS WE CAN INFLUENCE AND IMPACT, OR THAT WE CAN AT LEAST CHOOSE OUR RESPONSE TO:

- **Life experiences:** Childhood experiences, both positive and negative, have profound effects on our character, personality and emotions as we mature into adulthood. Because boys are encouraged to 'man up', act tough, stay in control and take what life throws at them – and actively discouraged from showing their softer side – as adults, they may find it difficult to seek support when they're struggling with something, especially their mental health and wellbeing.

- **Social and cultural influences:** Compared with women, men are more likely to eat an unhealthy diet, be overweight, drink excessive levels of alcohol, misuse drugs and be involved in an accident.

  And poor physical health among men can have a corresponding impact on their mental health. Men also tend to socialize differently to women, with fewer close relationships, which means that if they're struggling with their mental health, they have fewer people to rely on or to encourage them to get support. Because men tend to focus on work relationships, they can feel particularly unsupported if a problem occurs at work – for instance, conflict with colleagues or their line manager.

- **The impact of the workplace:** There is a great deal of pressure on men. Even though society is changing (which is good news) the majority of men continue to earn more than women and are more likely to occupy senior positions within an organization. Men are also twice as likely as women to work full-time and have a poor work-life balance, putting in inordinately long hours. They are also more likely to have the role as the main 'breadwinner' within a household.

Because work is so central to a man's life, when it is unsatisfying, disengaging or uncertain, it can be a significant source of mental distress and can impact the mental health of their family and those close to them.

Redundancy can also have an especially big impact on men, with their sense of purpose and contribution to their family and society more widely being questioned if they lose their job.

The reality is that men just aren't accessing help for mental health issues at an early stage which, of course, means that mental health problems are likely to last longer and go deeper. This will certainly change as work being undertaken by government, employers, charities and mental health campaigners cascades down to those who need help and awareness most urgently.

THE STIGMA THAT COMES WITH MENTAL HEALTH

Sadly, whether we like it or not, there is a stigma around mental health.

The stereotypes associated with men, in particular, being expected to act tough – to be 'real men' without 'soft emotions' – contribute significantly to the stigma attached to mental health problems and stop people from reaching out for help when their mental health is at risk.

The stigma around mental health can create the fear of being judged or discriminated against. This can discourage you from talking about your mental health and seeking support. As a result, it can feel impossible to talk with anyone about how you're feeling. Consequently, hiding your problem and hoping that it will go away really does seem like the easiest – or perhaps the only – option.

A poll conducted by the 'Time to Change' campaign (2015)[2] revealed that the stigma and discrimination individuals with a mental health problem face is often worse than the illness itself. In the study, 60% of respondents said that these negative reactions were as or more damaging than the symptoms of their problem, while 35% said that stigma had made them give up on their ambitions, hopes and dreams for their life. The poll also found that nearly half of people questioned (49%) felt uncomfortable talking with their employer about their mental health.

Unfortunately, this stigma won't go away overnight. But things are changing.

Celebrities, influencers and the younger members of the British Royal Family are proactively talking about and raising awareness of mental health issues. They're highlighting the importance of talking and seeking help, demonstrating that we are all in the same boat when it comes to potentially being affected by mental health problems.

Employers are also undertaking initiatives to promote positive mental health and educating their employees. Apart from simply being the right thing to do, it makes business sense for an organization to create a culture where employees feel able to talk openly – especially about their mental and physical health – and seek support without being judged or discriminated against.

Looking at the UK, initiatives like the mental health charity Mind's 'Time to Change' campaign are working hard to end the stigma and discrimination faced by those who experience mental health problems. Since the campaign began in 2007, Mind reports an improvement of 8.3% in public attitudes towards people with mental health problems.

Clearly, changes happening in the wider world don't always feel like they apply to daily life. Regardless of all the good work being done to eliminate the stigma associated with mental health problems, your reality might be very different.

But it's an undisputable fact that mental health problems can affect anyone, and there are people and organizations who can and will help you. You have nothing to be ashamed of.

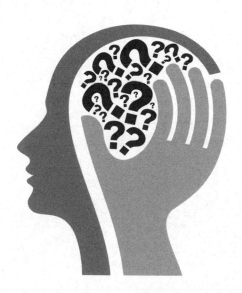

PART 2

TAKING CHARGE OF YOUR MENTAL HEALTH

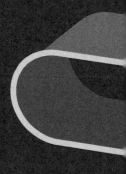

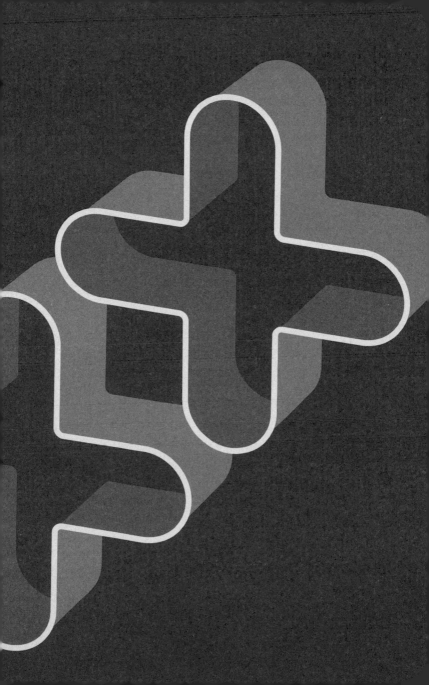

NURTURING OUR SELF-AWARENESS

Self-awareness is one of the cornerstones of emotional intelligence – that is the ability to recognize our own emotions, as well as those of those around us, using this knowledge to distinguish between different feelings and what they mean, and ultimately using this information to guide our behaviour, reactions and thinking.

As such, self-awareness is perhaps one of the most important characteristics required to nurture and develop in order to take charge of your mental health and wellbeing.

It is the conscious knowledge of ourselves, including our character, beliefs, desires, qualities, motivations and feelings. Having a good sense and understanding of each of these aspects can significantly benefit our feelings of engagement, success, satisfaction and contentment in our home and work lives.

Most of us have based our education and career decisions on what we've seen or picked up from those around us. But as we mature and grow, these actions and choices may no longer suit our current character, desires and preferences. This is where self-awareness can help identify alternative options that may be better suited to our individual preferences.

There are many tests that can help us identify and understand our character in more depth, including psychometric tests, coaching tools and self-reflection techniques. Having an enhanced understanding of ourselves has a wide-ranging positive impact on our working lives, contributing to:

- Understanding ours and other people's emotions more clearly

- Improving communication skills, encouraging workplace interactions, including looking at 'blind spots' that are outside of our immediate awareness

- Enhancing leadership skills, which can increase our performance at work

- Increasing job satisfaction by concentrating on the roles, responsibilities and tasks that motivate us

- Maximizing career development opportunities

To nurture self-awareness, it is useful to gather formal or informal feedback from those around us, to learn about ourselves and the impact we and our behaviour have on others.

Self-awareness provides the opportunity to think about how we interact and influence others, allowing us to adapt our behaviour and respond to different people and situations so that we can sustain our mental health and wellbeing.

"I had a mental health wobble over seven years ago which resulted in four months off work. My first steps to recovery were understanding what I can do to change. I stopped listening to the voices in my head and read the signals that told me I was about to have a wobble and talked with my wife when I was struggling. But the best thing was replacing alcohol with buying a dog! I have now found mindfulness to switch off those voices, I got fit and I have worked out how to avoid getting into those busy hectic bubbles, whether it be work, family or friends."

SELF-ESTEEM AND MENTAL HEALTH

Self-esteem reflects how much you value yourself, how you look after yourself and how you relate to others. When you are struggling to achieve positive mental health, it is highly likely that your self-esteem will suffer too.

"When my self-esteem is low, my mental health deteriorates. I take each day as it comes and I try to keep focused on things I can look forward to in the future."

Although self-esteem will build up over time and can be impacted by others – including your partner, parents, siblings and relatives, friends, work associates and manager – there are a few things you can do to build and develop it.

- **Understand the impact of change:** Self-esteem can be impacted by the way that you react and respond to change. Developing a positive outlook on change and being realistic about the influence you can have on an outcome contributes to preserving and protecting your self-esteem.

- **Look after your physical and mental health:** Good physical and mental health will help you cope with the stress and pressure that life throws at us. Exercising regularly, eating well, drinking enough water and getting plenty of rest and sleep will ensure that you hold yourself and your wellbeing in high regard.

- **Make some time for fun:** By engaging in fun and pleasurable pastimes, activities and experiences, you show yourself that you value your happiness, effectively increasing your sense of self-esteem.

- **Invest in your relationships:** Think about how much you expect of yourself when it comes to the relationships that are most important. What do you expect from other people, and what do you do to make sure that the time, emotion and energy you invest in relationships has a positive influence on your self-esteem?

- **Treat yourself properly:** Do you celebrate your positive characteristics and achievements, or do you focus on the negatives? Try to avoid people and situations that will negatively impact your self-esteem and ultimately bring you down. You could also keep a gratitude diary and note down regularly what you feel thankful for.

- **Take responsibility for your happiness:** Accept that you are in control of your destiny and that you have the power to build self-esteem. Don't wait for others to build you up or knock you down – take responsibility.

You can talk to a trusted friend or a professional about your self-esteem and what you can do to ensure it's as strong and resilient as it can be, so that it contributes to positive mental health.

"There is a huge link between self-esteem and mental health and when things are not going well, low self-esteem and feelings of not being good enough weaken my mental health. Fighting this with the knowledge that my feelings are normal and not beating myself up over things that I cannot change results in these feelings being short-lived and brushed off before they have negative effects."

THE LINK BETWEEN RESILIENCE AND MENTAL HEALTH

Resilience is our intuitive capacity to turn adversity into possibility – it's our 'bounce-back-ability' and what protects us from the setbacks that life throws at us. Emotional resilience is our attitude and response to the people, places and things that we face in our personal and working lives.

Essentially, resilience is the ability to deal with life as it is, not as you might want it to be. It's about adopting a learning approach to setbacks, seeing how we can learn from them and not letting them define us. In fact, a common feature of people who lack resilience is not only the stress and anxiety they suffer when faced with obstacles and upheavals, but also the length of time and effort it takes them to get over that stress and anxiety.

Things that make us less resilient as individuals can include factors relating to our upbringing, unresolved conflicts or simply the fact that we were born with certain sensitivities to different kinds of stress and pressure. Regardless of these, there are a number of factors that can erode our emotional resilience and impact our mental health and wellbeing:

- **Highly stressful or traumatic events:** People who have been involved in traumatic events can find that they're less resilient to future shocks.

- **Experiencing several stressful events at the same time:** Going through more than one significant life event or change at the same time tends to make people feel vulnerable. For example, financial difficulties, the threat of redundancy and the breakdown of a significant relationship happening together will have a hugely detrimental impact on a person's psychological wellbeing.

- **Experiencing stress over a long period of time:** When left unaddressed, cumulative stress can be as damaging as a one-off trauma. When someone is exposed to emotional pressure over and over again, their capacity to process it will eventually decline if the stress and its causes aren't dealt with.

- **Lack of control:** This can have a particularly damaging impact in the workplace. We are all given tasks we might not necessarily like or ask for, but those who have no choice over factors such as their pace of work or work patterns – or who aren't encouraged to use their skills or initiative at work – can feel worn down quite quickly.

- **Lack of social support:** Social support is a key factor in boosting resilience, and individuals without friends or partners (especially men) are at a greater risk than those with an established social support network.

When faced with one or a combination of these factors and situations, we can become deeply affected by stress. And should this happen, performance at work, decision-making, mood and behaviour, and mental health can all deteriorate.

"Taking a step out of my comfort zone and trying new things helped build my resilience, it was scary and sometimes embarrassing, but it all added to what I can deal with and offer."

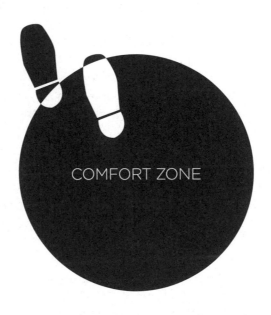

COMFORT ZONE

STEPS TO BECOMING MORE RESILIENT

In becoming more resilient it's important to nurture and develop behaviours that enable you to better manage pressure and promote physical and mental wellbeing. Here are a few suggestions on the steps you can take to become more resilient.

- **Build your inner toughness:** This includes the confidence to believe that you will survive and come through hard times, nurturing a sense of optimism and engagement with life and work.

- **Make sure you practice supportive thinking:** This is the ability to think in a reflective and rational way, noticing the effect of your thoughts on your own wellbeing, as well as listening to others and allowing and accommodating for differences in your personality and performance.

- **Find solutions:** Build the capacity to identify problems, set goals and apply solutions to maintain your mental and physical effectiveness in the face of possible difficulties or outcomes.

- **Create connections:** Be aware of the need for emotional support and think about how you can access this, making the most of feedback and support from a range of different people and sources, including co-workers and mentors.

- **Self-regulate your emotions:** Find a way to return to a calm state after feeling upset or emotional. Think about and analyse the potential consequences of your actions and your ability to switch off and refresh.

- **Implement positive life habits:** Commit to eating regularly and eating well, as well as relaxing and making time to refresh your mind and body.

Combined with these steps, there are some strategies that you can employ to deal with the triggers that impact our ability to cope:

- **Identify your vulnerabilities:** Before creating strategies that can boost resilience, you need to know what you are up against. Try to become more emotionally aware, noting the times and situations when you feel stressed and overwhelmed to better understand your trigger points and create strategies to address them. This is the opposite to being like an ostrich, which sticks its head in the ground and ignores what's going on around it.

- **Challenge negative thoughts:** It is easy to let pessimism become a habit. But fortunately, like any habit, this can be changed with a bit of effort and a lot of perseverance. As with identifying vulnerabilities, make note of any negative thoughts, challenge yourself when they are recognized and reflect on how reasonable they are. Is there a way to reframe your thinking and consider your thoughts in a more positive and logical way?

- **Accept what you can't change:** If you are resilient you will understand that a situation, good or bad, has to be accepted before it can be changed. Sitting in silence for a few minutes each day, breathing steadily and simply observing your thoughts and emotions is a great way to cultivate acceptance and boost resilience.

- **Get some exercise:** Regular exercise works off stress hormones, promotes a sense of positive wellbeing and prepares you for the next challenge. If you find it hard to get a regular exercise programme going, start small with a regular walk during your lunch break. Even a little bit of exercise will make all the difference. In fact, even having a lunch break and getting out and about away from a sedentary, desk-based lifestyle is a great start.

- **Make sure you have social support:** Studies on resilience often show that social support is vital to maintaining solid emotional resilience. If you have good friends or colleagues to talk to, reach out to them regularly. If you feel deeply cut off and isolated from those around you, it could be time to get a bit of outside help.

- **Create some positive habits:** Whether it's exercising, spending time with friends and loved ones, or just making time for quiet reflection, it gets a lot easier to do something once it becomes a habit. Regularly setting aside short periods of time for resilience-boosting activities saves a lot of mental and physical energy and will make a dramatic difference to your life in the long term.

"As easy and as strong the pull is to retreat from people, I have found that being around others boosts your mental wellbeing."

GETTING A GOOD NIGHT'S SLEEP

Sleep is perhaps the biggest contributor to living better and a key factor in taking charge of your mental health. The amount of sleep that we need varies for each individual, but on average adults sleep for about seven and a half hours a night. If you do lose a few nights' sleep, it's not the end of the world. Although you might feel tired and grumpy, it will not always affect your overall mental health and performance levels.

But when things are tough, you're stressed and your mental health is taking a bashing, it can be difficult to get a good night's sleep. When you're not sleeping well and getting insufficient rest, you feel weary, irritable and less able to tackle stressful situations. And when you start to feel like you can't cope, you enter into a negative cycle of feeling stressed about not sleeping, which inevitably leads to more sleepless nights.

Most of us are affected by insomnia at some point in our lives – in fact, one in three of us will suffer from this.[3] It happens most often when we're feeling stressed or under pressure.

The underlying physiological cause is higher levels of adrenalin in our bodies, which makes it difficult to relax and interrupts our usual sleep patterns.

Of course, mental health struggles aren't the only reason that you might not be sleeping. For example, are you taking any new medication? Have you drunk more caffeine or alcohol than you usually do, or done so at a different time of day? Is your bedroom too hot or too cold? Are your neighbours being noisier than usual?

Sleep patterns change as we get older. We tend to become lighter sleepers and our sleep is more easily interrupted, so it's worth thinking whether this could apply to you.

The good news is that there are things you can do to help ensure a good night's sleep.

HERE ARE JUST A FEW OF THE OPTIONS:

+

- Establish a daily bed time regardless of whether you feel tired or not

- Keep your bed for sleep. Don't watch TV, eat or discuss issues that won't get resolved right before bedtime

- Make an effort to relax before you go to bed – maybe read a book, listen to music or take a bath

- Cut out intake of caffeine or alcohol a few hours before bed and avoid having a heavy meal or spicy food at a late hour

- If you haven't fallen asleep after half an hour, go to another room and do something undemanding, such as reading or ironing for 10 or 15 minutes, and then try again. But remember that even stretching out and relaxing will give you some benefits, which is much better than tossing and turning for hours!

- Redirect your thinking by using distraction exercises to divert your brain's nervous energy. These can include remembering the names of football teams, counties or cities, and so on. It's essentially the old idea of 'counting sheep'

If nothing is working and you have regular sleepless nights, it's probably time to visit your doctor or other health professional.

Along with insomnia there are other sleep problems – such as sleep apnoea or restless leg syndrome, as well as other underlying medical issues like dealing with pain management – that can impact your sleep patterns and need to get sorted out.

"I have a fairly good and regular bedtime routine and attempt to be in bed at the same time every night. I have suffered from insomnia for a number of years, but since being in a stable and loving relationship this has much improved. Motherhood has also helped me to deal with a lack of sleep in a better way, and now I'm used to having disrupted sleep but being able to cope!"

EATING FOR POSITIVE MENTAL HEALTH

What we eat and how we eat it can have a massive impact on both our mental and physical health.

When we eat well, it's likely that we'll think more clearly, be in a better mood and have more positive energy, which is also very good for our physical health.

We need a healthy balanced diet to help maintain good mental and physical health, which is something we can achieve by incorporating the following elements:

- **Get your 'five a day':** Get the minerals, vitamins and fibre you need to maintain your physical and mental health from fruit and vegetables. Try to eat at least five different fruits and vegetables, and whether they're fresh, frozen, dried or tinned, they all count towards your target.

- **Incorporate the right fats into your diet:** Our bodies, and particularly our brains, need fatty acids, such as omega-3 and omega-6 to keep them thriving. Healthy fats can be obtained from oily fish like mackerel and tuna, poultry, eggs, nuts and seeds, olive and sunflower oils and dairy products such as yoghurt, cheese and milk.

- **Base your meals on higher fibre starchy foods:** These include potatoes, bread, rice and pasta and should make up about one third of what you eat. Wholegrain and wholemeal varieties of starchy foods like brown rice, whole-wheat pasta and wholemeal bread contain more fibre, vitamins and minerals.

- **Get some protein on your plate:** Milk and dairy foods such as cheese and yoghurt are good sources of protein, as well as containing calcium to keep bones healthy. Protein can also be found in beans, pulses, fish, eggs and meat.

- **Eat less saturated fat, sugar and salt:** Eating too much saturated fat can increase the amount of cholesterol in the blood, which can increase your risk of developing heart disease. Combined with this, consuming food and drink with high levels of sugar can contribute to obesity and tooth decay. And too much salt in your diet raises blood pressure, increasing the risks of having heart disease or stroke.

- **Watch how much caffeine you have:** As a stimulant, caffeine can offer a quick energy boost but one which is followed by a depressed feeling and even anxiety. It can disturb sleep patterns and lead to withdrawal symptoms and if that's the case cut it out quickly.

As well as watching what you eat as part of a balanced diet, how you plan meals and eat food can have a significant impact on your health. Here is some advice to incorporate into your plans to eat for positive mental health:

- **Plan ahead:** Whether it's creating a meal plan for the week ahead or batch cooking some healthy meals for the freezer, so you've always got a well-balanced meal to hand. Planning will help you to feel in control of your diet.

- **Keep a food diary:** Keeping a record of what you eat, when you eat it and how it makes you feel can help you monitor if some foods make you feel better or worse.

- **Try to eat regularly:** Creating a routine for your meals – and not being tempted to skip meals – can help to maintain your mood, energy and blood sugar levels, as well as giving a structure to your day.

- **If you need to snack, make them healthy:** Incorporating healthy snacks into your meal planning can help you avoid feeling irritable or tired. Avoiding sweets biscuits, sugary drinks and alcohol will stop your blood sugar rising and falling rapidly and help you stay more in control.

- **Consider how your food affects your mood:** Incorporating slow-release energy foods, such as protein, nuts, seeds, oats and whole grains can help to maintain energy and blood sugar levels.

- **Slow down and take time:** Avoid the temptation to eat and run, but rather setting the dining table and sitting down to eat slowly will have a positive influence on your mental health. Focus on the quality, taste and enjoyment of food to help you feel satisfied.

As with many of the factors that influence our mental health, there is help out there. If you need support with your diet and its impact on your mental or physical health, reach out to your doctor or a registered dietician who are well placed to help you find the right information and support.

"My diet affects my mental health massively. Sometimes I get caught up in a vicious circle of feeling anxious, stress eating and then feeling anxious as I am overweight and not having the right nutrients I require. When I eat healthily, I feel better in myself both mentally and physically."

WATER, HYDRATION AND YOUR MENTAL HEALTH

As well as being essential for life, water and staying hydrated is essential for good mental health.

Not drinking enough water affects concentration and the ability to think clearly and physically. We might get a headache or feel light-headed, have a dry mouth, feel tired and a bit sick. And often, by the time we feel thirsty we're already dehydrated and need to grab a drink!

We're told that drinking about eight glasses of water – that's about two litres – is our goal when it comes to being properly hydrated, but if you're exercising or in a particularly hot environment, you probably need to increase this amount.

If you haven't quite mastered the art of watering your mental health, there are a few things you can do to make sure that you're drinking enough and staying hydrated:

- If you're not keen on the taste of water, why not try herbal or fruit tea, sugar-free cordial or diluted fruit juice or even put a slice of lemon, lime, orange or cucumber in your water to give it some flavour

- Keep a bottle of water close with you during the day and keep sipping

- If you keep forgetting to drink, set a reminder on your phone or calendar or pop a note on your desk or fridge

Drinking the right drink is also important: caffeinated tea and coffee, sugary drinks and alcohol do not hydrate you and shouldn't be counted towards your daily water intake.

"I know when I haven't drunk enough water because I find that my concentration is slipping and I'll become a bit forgetful. I'm definitely more focused when I drink water regularly throughout the day."

ALCOHOL AND MENTAL HEALTH

Approximately 24% of adults in England and Scotland regularly drink over the Chief Medical Officer's guidelines,[4] which increases their long-term risk of becoming ill, and even more (27%) drinkers in Great Britain binge drink on their heaviest drinking days.[5]

It's easy for these drinking habits to transform our mental health and whilst alcohol can have a temporary positive impact on our mood and perceived levels of happiness, it can have a hugely negative impact on our mental health in the longer term.

Alcohol use and misuse is linked to a wide range of mental health issues, including depression, insomnia, anxiety and it's even a factor in suicide rates. Ultimately, alcohol is a depressant and it changes the chemical balance of the brain. The more we drink, the more damage we can do and if we drink heavily and regularly we start to develop symptoms of depression. In fact, people who experience anxiety or depression are more likely to be heavy or problem drinkers.[6]

Alongside contributing to feelings of depression, alcohol can affect mental health in a number of other ways:

- **Memory loss:** Alcohol slows down the processes in the brain, which means we can forget the things we get up to when drunk. Frequently drinking too much can cause more permanent damage to the brain.

- **Suicide and self-harm:** Research shows that more than half of people admitted to hospital because of deliberate self-harm and injury confessed to drinking immediately before or while they'd done it.[7]

- **Relationship breakdown:** Although alcohol can help to build relationships, it can also lead to arguments and bad behaviour that contributes to relationship breakdown.

- **Poor sleeping habits:** Whilst some people claim to sleep better when they've had a drink or two, alcohol disrupts the regular sleep cycle so we feel tired, irritable and dehydrated the following day, often craving unhealthy foods.

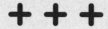

SOME POSITIVE STEPS TO TAKE WHEN ALCOHOL IS AFFECTING YOUR MENTAL HEALTH:

- If you're drinking to manage stress, try something different such as going for a walk or taking an exercise class to reduce stress levels. And if you're drinking to mask a specific problem, consider trying to talk with a friend, relative, counsellor or healthcare professional about it

- Be a more mindful drinker, taking time to think why you're having a drink. Is it to mask a feeling? Or is it a habit? You could also keep an honest record of how much you're drinking in a week; the results will show if you have a problem

- Review if you're drinking every day and if you are, why? Can you incorporate a few alcohol-free days into your schedule to help ensure you're not becoming addicted? Or offer to drive if you're going out socially so you're not tempted to have a drink?

"I used to drink quite a lot of alcohol and used it as a coping strategy for my poor mental health. I dealt with this through local support groups and the support of my family, which made the biggest impact. I still drink alcohol but now I only drink at weekends which gives me something to look forward to as it's sociable rather than me drinking frequently on my own."

Our mental health, just like our physical health, is impacted by a range of factors.

MOVEMENT, EXERCISE AND MENTAL HEALTH

It's no secret that regular exercise is good for our bodies, but it's easy to forget that it's also a fantastic way to keep our minds in tip top shape, improving our wellbeing and helping to overcome some of the most common mental health challenges and problems.

Even the smallest amount of activity can start to improve your mood; beginning with a walk around the block and extending this out to a longer walk every few days as your stamina, motivation and energy levels begin to build.

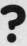

Did you know that about one-third of adults in England are damaging their health because of a lack of physical activity?

Or that one in four women and one in five men in England are defined as inactive because they're doing less than 30 minutes of moderate physical activity every week?[8]

As you start to move more, you'll begin to feel more energetic throughout the day, more relaxed and generally more positive about yourself and your life. You'll also start to see some of the other mental health benefits of exercise:

- It can help to improve concentration and memory, as well as stimulating the growth of new brain cells

- It can help you to sleep better and build a routine, particularly by incorporating regular exercise into your life and making exercise a positive habit

- It relieves tension and stress and boosts wellbeing through the release of endorphins, those fabulous chemicals in your brain that make you feel good

- It provides a distraction to how you're feeling, helping to break a cycle of negative thinking and giving you something different to focus on

As well as getting in the right 'head space' for wanting to move more and incorporate some exercise and physical activity into your life, there is plenty you can do to make sure that you're ready to move and stay motivated.

- **Do what you enjoy:** It sounds great to have a goal of running a marathon or completing a triathlon, but that type of endurance activity isn't for everyone. Think about what activity makes you happy – it might be walking the dog, jogging with a friend, gardening, swimming, playing Frisbee or soccer with your children or friends, taking a class at a local gym or even walking around a local shopping centre. The key is to find something that you enjoy and once you've started moving, challenge yourself to do something new and different.

- **Reward your achievements:** As well as improving your mental health, you might want to think about a reward or treat for achievements. It could be a bath, a massage, a meal with your partner or a 15-minute nap on the sofa, something that acknowledges the investment you're making in your physical and mental health.

- **Remember you don't have to do it alone!:** Making exercise a social activity, whether with friends, family or a class, is a great way to keep motivated. It can help to have someone that encourages you out of the door on the days when you don't feel like exercising, as well as having someone to celebrate achievements with.

- **Incorporate activity into your daily life:** You could get off the bus or train one stop ahead of your destination and walk the rest of the way, take the stairs rather than the lift or escalator, set a reminder to stand up regularly throughout the day. Think about how you can add extra activities into your regular routine to keep your motivation levels high.

"The best exercise for my mental health is walking; this supports my mindfulness practice and allows me to be outdoors where I feel most at ease. This is important as I know when I feel at my most anxious, going for a walk is a great coping mechanism and doing it regularly helps me maintain a healthy mind."

BREAKING DOWN THE BARRIERS THAT STOP US BEING ACTIVE

We can be our own worst enemies when it comes to incorporating movement and exercise as a regular part of our lives. Too often we tell ourselves that we can't or shouldn't do something that deep down we know will be good for us.

Fortunately, some of the most common barriers that we put in place to stop ourselves from getting active can be relatively easily overcome.

- **I'm too tired to exercise ...** It's easy to believe that when you're stressed and anxious, exercise will make you feel more tired and zap any energy that you have. That's just not the case. Regular exercise will boost your energy levels and start to reduce the feelings of weariness and lethargy that you're experiencing.

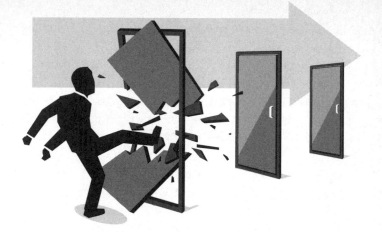

- **I'm too unfit, there's just no point ...** We all have to start somewhere and even if you've not done any exercise for years, it's not too late to start now. Even the smallest changes, such as parking as far away from the shops or office as possible to get in a few more steps, will have a positive impact on how you feel.

- **I hate exercise ...** Fortunately exercise isn't all about pounding a treadmill or bouncing around in an aerobics class. There are loads of ways to increase your physical activity levels and there's definitely something for everyone, it just takes a moment or two to decide what works for you. Gardening, dancing, walking, swimming, pilates, yoga, cycling, weight training, tennis, hiking, martial arts. Take a moment and think what you might like to do.

- **I haven't got time ...** You might be a busy person, but it's a case of simply making the time. If you've reached the point where you recognize that exercise and activity is something that you need to do, then prioritize it in your schedule. Be realistic, how much time do you spend sat on the sofa watching TV or scrolling through social media? There's a fair chance you could invest this time better – start with 10 or 15 minutes a day.

- **It's not worth it, I'm a lost cause ...** We can be our own worst critics when it comes to positive body image and how we feel about ourselves. It's important to accept that you're not on your own, but you are in control. Take a look at all the options available and find a class, a trainer or an activity that will help reassure you that you're not alone. There are others who will understand how you feel and support you to make a change.

- **It's going to hurt too much ...** If you're in pain because of a physical illness or condition, you should be able to get some advice and information from your healthcare professional about the type of activity that is best suited to you. Rather than ignore the pain or let it stop you from doing what you want to do, try low impact activities such as swimming, or try to do more regular and frequent exercise for shorter periods of time.

SAYING 'STOP' TO BULLYING AND HARASSMENT

Bullying and harassment – whether it's being done in a sneaky or more open way – can happen at any point in life, from school to work and every social interaction in between.

A bully is someone who misuses their power, position or knowledge to criticise, humiliate and destroy another person's competence, confidence, integrity and effectiveness. And when it comes to your mental health, bullying will have a massive impact, messing with your head and making you feel anxious, stressed and depressed.

Harassment, in distinct contrast to bullying, is any inappropriate or unwanted behaviour that could reasonably be perceived by the direct recipient (or any other person) as affecting their dignity, self-respect and self-esteem.

This could include suggestive remarks and gestures, comments, jokes or banter that focuses on age, creed, disability, nationality, race, sex, sexual orientation, family status, religion or any other personal characteristic. It can be a one-off event or a series of actions that are carried out by an individual or a group of people.

Bullying and harassment hugely impact mental health and are likely to lead to a range of challenging emotions and feelings. They leave people:

- Anxious and worried, as well as sad and tearful
- Angry and stressed
- Worthless and unloved
- Helpless and hopeless
- Physically sick
- At risk of self-harm
- Struggling to concentrate
- Wanting to hide from social and work interactions
- Losing appetite, or turning to comfort eating
- Relying on drugs or alcohol to cope
- Having trouble sleeping and relaxing
- Experiencing flashbacks and nightmares

Bullying isn't acceptable at any level, or in any social or work situation. No one has the right to make another feel ashamed, frightened or lonely. If you are being bullied, you have the power to make it stop, despite what the bully might be telling you, and there are people and organizations that are ready, willing and able to help you.

- Talk to your doctor about what you are going through and how it is making you feel, especially if you are struggling with thoughts of self-harm, suicide, depression or anxiety as a result of the bullying or harassment. Make notes before your appointment so you remember all the symptoms that you are experiencing

- If your employer has an Employee Assistance Programme (EAP), they are on hand at any time to talk to you about what's been happening, in a safe, confidential and non-judgemental environment

- Other specialist organizations can also help you avoid future instances of bullying and harassment

Talking with a professional about what has happened can help you to better understand, for example, your company's bullying and harassment policy and help you to weigh up the pros and cons of raising a complaint rather than challenging the bully informally.

Beyond reaching out for professional help, there are also things you can do to take care of yourself:

- Look after your physical wellbeing: eat well, drink lots of water, avoid alcohol and drugs and maintain a regular exercise programme

- Find time to relax and take a break: practice relaxation techniques and try some breathing exercises. Despite what is happening to you, by being relaxed you will be in the best mindset to deal with the perpetrators

- Record what's been happening – keep a diary of what has been happening, jotting down incidents, dates and times on paper or on your smartphone or computer. This will help you build a timeline of events and record the names of any witnesses who might be able to support you in the future, especially if you make a formal complaint or report

Sadly, bullying and harassment do take place and people behave in ways that are, without beating around the bush, totally unacceptable. But remember, although it might not feel like it, you do have the power to stop what is happening to you, so please take action if this is something that you are suffering from.

WHEN LONELINESS BECOMES A MENTAL HEALTH PROBLEM

Whilst loneliness is not in itself a mental health problem, the two are very closely connected. Having a mental health problem can increase your chance of feeling lonely and isolated, and feeling all alone can have a negative impact on mental health.

We all have different social needs. Although most of us need some sort of social contact to maintain good mental health, some might be satisfied with a few close friends and others will desire a large group with lots of acquaintances. In some ways this is influenced by our personality, so an extrovert will feel the impact of isolation more acutely than an introvert.

Of course, it is important to recognize that being alone is not the same as being lonely, and if you're comfortable with your own company, there is nothing wrong with being on your own.

But if you are feeling lonely – perhaps because you don't see or talk to others very often or if, even though you're surrounded by people, you don't feel understood or cared for – there are some things you can do to cope and feel better.

- **Think about how you can meet and connect with new people**
  You could overcome loneliness by trying to meet new or different people. Maybe take a class, join a local group or volunteer for a charity or community organization.

  Or, if you're not quite ready to meet new people face-to-face, you could interact with others online. Although online engagement may help alleviate loneliness, it's important to be careful. For example, never share personal information like your home address or banking information. And, needless to say, you should always exercise caution if someone starts pushing to meet in person.

- **Talk to people around you about how you're feeling**
  Even if you have a lot of people around you, you may feel that they are not giving you the care, attention, responsiveness and consideration that you need. The best way to manage this, as hard as it might seem, is to open up and explain how you feel, perhaps suggesting how things could be different. There is every chance that they hadn't realized that their behaviour was impacting you in this way and that they are willing to change.

- **Don't expect things to change overnight**
  Changing the way that you interact with people, or meeting new people, won't happen overnight. It takes time, so don't feel the need to rush into anything.

When meeting new people, manage your expectations and don't expect full-blown interaction straight away. Take time to acclimatize to a new group or situation and observe what is happening. Then, you'll be able to choose the best time to jump in!

- **Resist the temptation to compare yourself to others**
  If you're comparing yourself to others on social media and dwelling on how they're feeling, what they're doing and what they have achieved, you are going to be disappointed. A social media post only tells one side of a story – too often projecting a carefully contrived, artificially upbeat, filtered and edited online persona – so don't take any of it too seriously, and perhaps think about spending less time on your favourite social media channels if you suspect that they are impacting negatively on your mental wellbeing.

It is also helpful to reflect on how your feelings of loneliness might be affecting your health. If they are making you feel upset, it will certainly impact your mental and physical health, so it's important to take action and make changes that will protect your overall wellbeing. Interestingly, research has shown that lacking social connections can be as damaging to our health as smoking 15 cigarettes a day.[9]

As mentioned earlier, the first and often most painful and challenging step is to recognize where you are. This is the springboard to taking action to improve the situation and how you feel, so be brave and make a change.

SOCIAL MEDIA AND MENTAL HEALTH

Social media is now an established part of our lives – 40% of the world's population reportedly uses it –[10] and whether it's Instagram, Facebook, Snapchat, Twitter or any other platform that encourages sharing life snippets and opinions as well as snooping on other people's lives, it seems that social media is here to stay.

Since it is now such an integral part of our day-to-day existence, it's only to be expected that social media can positively and negatively impact our mental health.

When it comes to positively influencing mental health, social media can be particularly useful. It can offer a great support system during difficult times, providing access to a whole host of professional experts, as well as those who have had direct and personal experience of issues being faced. Online communities can provide a great source of emotional support, offering a platform where questions that can't necessarily be asked out loud are funnelled. That contributes to reducing feelings of isolation or anxiety and effectively helps individuals to find the answers that can support mental health.

However, as good as it can be, there are a number of studies that point to the damage that social media can do to your mental health. Some studies have found a link between social media use and depression and anxiety and, particularly worryingly, an increased risk of suicide.[11]

Social media can encourage feelings of inadequacy regarding life and achievements. Researchers found that three out of every five Facebook and Twitter users felt that their own achievements were inadequate when compared with the posts of others, as well as making them feel jealous of other users.[12]

Another cause for concern is the link between sleep disruption caused by excessive mobile phone usage at night with depression and unhappiness.[13] People who spend the night checking social media are more likely to suffer from mood problems, including neuroticism and bipolar disorder, and consider themselves less happy and lonelier.

Social media can also actually make us feel more isolated than connected. A study of 7,000 people found that those who spend the most time on social media were more likely to report feeling social isolation, including a lack of a sense of social belonging, engagement with others and fulfilling relationships.[14]

With social media, it's far too easy to compare our lives with those of the people we follow. It's only human nature. But that's not healthy: one study found that regularly using Facebook could lead to symptoms of depression if the site triggered feelings of envy in the user.[15]

Another study pointed to people demonstrating psychological symptoms of withdrawal, including increased heart rate and blood pressure, as well as anxiety, when they stopped using social media and the internet.[16]

It's important to recognize how easy it is to become addicted to social media – not helped by the fact that it's such a core part of life today and that often the problem is not realized until it's too late – but by taking a step back and assessing your social media usage, it's easier to reflect on how it affects your mental health.

"I take a very realistic view of social media. Whilst I enjoy looking at it and catching up with my friends and family's activities, I am very mindful that the images and life portrayed on the internet are not always a true reflection of what lies behind the lens, and whilst other people's lives look rich with monetary ease and glossy homes and holidays, reading between the lines, life for these people is not all we are led to believe."

HELP YOURSELF TO MANAGE YOUR SOCIAL MEDIA USE

If you're spending too much time on social media and not enough in the real world, now might be the time to try to manage this addiction.

1. **Acknowledge that you've got a problem!**
   The first step, of course, to solving a problem is admitting that there is one.

   Are you checking your Facebook feed from the moment you wake up, or finding that you're taking a photo of every single thing you eat and posting it on Instagram? When out with a friend, do you find yourself constantly checking your social media accounts on your phone? Are you scrolling through your phone while you're sat on the sofa with your partner, supposedly watching television or listening to their day? Have you developed a 'fear of missing out' if you can't get to your phone to see what's been going on?

If you find yourself nodding in agreement in response to any of these questions, then it's a good moment to acknowledge you may have a problem.

2. **Remove the temptation from your home screen**
   Receiving push notifications for recent activity on social media platforms is just too tempting and can immediately encourage scrolling to see what is going on. By disabling push notifications you'll help to cut the time you spend online. You can also 'snooze' some of the traffic on news feeds by opting to temporarily stop seeing posts from some groups and pages.

3. **Reflect on what else you could be doing**
   As tempting as social media is, consider what you're really getting from it and the value it adds to your life. Could you be reading a book, watching a film, catching up with friends, taking up a new hobby or spending more time with your partner? Are you brave enough to put the phone down and do something different?

4. **Ask yourself how many social channels do you really need?**
   There always seems to be something new when it comes to social media such as new, enticing platforms. But do you really need another way to view a news feed? Reviewing the accounts that you have and resisting the lure of opening new accounts, however trendy, is a positive way to manage social media usage.

5. **Make your social media contributions matter**

Before posting your latest thoughts, take a moment to make your contribution matter. Is it really important and necessary to share? Who are you really talking to and, hand on heart, are they that interested? By thinking twice about posting you will better analyse your social media use and cut back on time spent on it.

6. **Nurture real-world relationships and experiences**

Today, it's second nature to take a photo of an experience or video your favourite song at a concert, rather than enjoying the moment in real time. How often do we really look back on these once captured and posted? How many people really watch them? So, if the answer is, 'not that many', why do we bother? Surely it's better to enjoy relationships and experiences in the real world?

7. **Are you brave enough to take a break?**

Maybe taking a break for a week seems like a really long, unmanageable, time. But how about taking a break from social media for an evening to start with and then a day? It'll still be there when you pop back on it and, surely, if it's really important news, your friends and family will pick up the phone or pop around to tell you what's happening? If not, then perhaps they need to read this book!

ACHIEVING A POSITIVE WORK/ LIFE BALANCE

A work/life balance is the amount of time and focus given to work compared with the other aspects of your life, whether that's your partner and family, hobbies, sport, voluntary work or more general home life.

When work and life are out of balance, you can suffer physically, emotionally and even financially and there's likely to be an impact on your relationships and performance. Putting too much emphasis on one part of life, such as work, can also lead to burnout and stress. Yet once a positive work/life balance is achieved and maintained, it's highly likely that your overall happiness, wellbeing and mental health will be improved.

Of course, work/life balance is unique to each individual and depends on the stage of life. But with the right tools in place to better manage it, you'll be able to adapt to the changes and challenges that life puts in the way.

The first positive step to achieve a better work/life balance is to reflect and consider your current professional and personal life demands. Once you have a deeper under-standing of the way your time and focus is divided and how you might like this to change, you can start to find a path to a better balance.

To reach this better balance, think about setting more re-alistic and achievable boundaries between your work and life priorities. Can your work day and working hours be better defined? Can you manage emails better and resist the temptation to check them out of hours?

Identify your priorities for work and life and set key goals to re-organize your time and meet these priorities. As part of this, you might want to think about what's urgent and what's important; often the two can get easily confused.

As well as meeting the demands that the various elements of your life can have, it's easy to lose sight of what's import-ant and instead try to fulfil commitments to and demands of others. Consider whether you have time to do something for yourself. Can you find time for regular breaks for your-self, whether it's for a walk around the block, to watch your favourite film or programme or to have dinner with friends?

Perhaps one of the key tricks to achieving a positive work/life balance is learning to say 'no'. It's not possible to do everything in one go, and you'll only put yourself under pressure by even attempting it.

"It took me a long time to develop a positive work/life balance. I love my job and hadn't realized how little time

I was spending at home. Taking a longer summer holiday when my daughter was six months old really gave me a jolt and made me realize that my priorities were out of shape. When I got back from holiday, I spoke to my manager who was incredibly supportive in helping me to set work/life balance goals and sending me reminders to make sure I was actually leaving the office!"

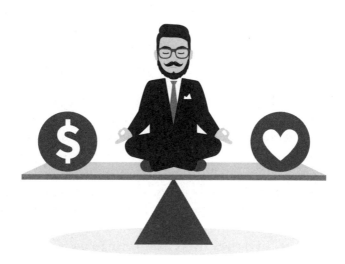

MINIMIZING THE IMPACT OF MONEY ON MENTAL HEALTH

Money and mental health have a very close relationship. Worrying about money will affect your mental health and poor mental health can make managing money very challenging. According to the Royal College of Psychiatrists, one in four people with a mental health problem is also in debt.[17]

Research by the Money and Mental Health Policy Institute found a clear link between financial difficulties and mental health, reporting that 41% of employees who identified themselves as 'financially comfortable' reported at least one sign of poor mental health.[18] This figure rises to 51% for people who say they're 'just about managing' and 67% for those 'in financial difficulty'.

This study also identified that an individual's ability to work is compromised because of financial worries, with people struggling to concentrate, losing sleep, lacking motivation and feeling under pressure.

Debt and money worries can make many aspects of life feel out of control. If financial issues are affecting your mental health – or, just as easily, vice versa – there are positive steps that can improve your financial wellbeing and minimize the impact that money issues have on your mental health.

- **Think about how your mental health affects your money management**
  How do you spend money? Why do you spend it on what you do? For example, do you spend money to make yourself feel better when things are tough? Or have you had to take time off work, which has affected your income?

  Is there a part of managing your money that affects your mental health? For example, do you get anxious when you open a letter from the bank or a credit card company? Or are you struggling with debt, but feel unable to pick up the phone to talk with someone about it?

  Having a better understanding of your behaviour when it comes to money will help you to identify the best things to do to get back on track.

- **Talk to someone you trust about the situation you find yourself in**
  Although it can be hard to start a conversation about money (and how it's making you feel), it can be helpful to talk with someone you trust, whether it's a friend, a family member, your doctor or another health professional.

Give some consideration to the impact that your money problems are or could be having on your relationships. It can be hard to talk to a partner about money or debt issues, and you might find it hard to open up to them if you need to rely on them for financial support whilst you are struggling with your mental health.

- **Get your paperwork in order**
  Find a regular time to look at account statements, bills and tax notices so you're on top of what is happening and there aren't any surprises waiting for you. It is good practice to keep all financial paperwork and important documents together, so that if you need to check something, you can go straight to what you need.

  Procrastination is definitely a potential problem here; it's tempting to put off working through tedious paperwork so a 'little and often' approach will help avoid an unmanageable crunch down the road. However, if your paperwork is a mess, it pays to get a handle on it today so that it will be better next time.

- **Make the most of the experts that are out there**
  If you are finding it hard to manage your money and it's affecting your day-to-day life and mental health, seek advice from an expert. This could be an advisor at your bank, a debt management charity or your EAP helpline, which can direct you to someone who can help you work through the situation.

There are also fabulous (and freely accessible) websites, such as MoneySavingExpert.com which has information, action plans, advice and tips, as well as forums where you can learn from the experiences and successes of other people who have been in the same position.

It is easy to underestimate just how much money worries can affect your mood, behaviour, performance at work and overall wellbeing, so it's something best tackled as soon as it's recognized that money – or a lack of it – is affecting your mental health.

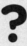

On a practical level, why not consider some of these simple tactics to help with day-to-day money management?

- Recognize you have an issue with money – it's very common, many people do – but accept that by sorting out these issue(s) your mental health will improve

- Avoid the temptation of spending and take positive action to do something else. Go for a walk, chat with a friend or clean out a cupboard at home, perhaps?

- De-register your credit or debit card details from online stores that you purchase from. This makes impulse purchases more difficult if temptation does strike

- Use online banking and web chat services if you find it hard to talk with your bank face-to-face or on the phone about money troubles. Most banks have a policy to help customers who proactively come forward with financial worries and they will be supportive

- If you are self-employed, get strict with saving for tax that you'll owe at some point down the line, perhaps by putting it in a different account so you don't get a false sense of security with your bank account balance

"You can only control the things within your power. Let go of the things that you can't influence as they will never change. You can only deal with one issue at a time, especially related to money, so make a list and work your way through it. Visual lists of what you have to do are a lot easier to comprehend and manage than the feeling of dread in your mind because there's so much going on. There is always someone to help, whether it be family, friends or something more established."

GAMBLING AND MENTAL HEALTH

Gambling is a popular pastime for many people. In itself it's not really a problem, offering us an exciting way to get a buzz and an adrenaline rush. When gambling is a positive pastime, it's likely that:

- We have thought about how much we can afford to lose and have set a budget. When we've reached our limits, we are prepared to walk away

- Gambling isn't a habit and we can limit the amount of time devoted to it

- We aren't tempted by high-risk forms of gambling where there is a danger of losing a lot of money very quickly

- We can quit when we're ahead and aren't enticed to chase the next big win

Unfortunately for some, gambling can quickly and easily become a serious problem that impacts their mental health, general wellbeing and personal finances.

"Gambling has made me so depressed and fed up that I'm not really talking to anyone and distancing myself further from people at work. I realize how stupid I've been but that's what gambling addiction does to me and I don't know how I can get over this. I feel so depressed right now and unsure what to do. With my debts I just don't see a way out."

Problem gambling, as defined by the Royal College of Psychiatrists, is gambling that "disrupts or damages personal, family or recreational pursuits" and affects about nine people in every 1,000.[19] That said, a further 70 people in every 1,000 gamble at risky levels which could become a problem in the future.

The college goes on to report that problem gamblers are more likely to suffer from low self-esteem, develop stress-related disorders, become anxious, have poor sleep and appetite, to develop a substance misuse problem and to suffer from depression.

A recent study also indicated that problem gamblers were 15 times more likely to commit suicide.[20]

**IF YOU SUSPECT THAT YOU MIGHT
HAVE A GAMBLING PROBLEM,
TAKE A FEW MOMENTS TO CONSIDER
THE ANSWER TO THESE QUESTIONS:**

Does the thought of gambling
make you unhappy?

Is it interfering with your sleep
or general concentration?

Do you gamble to distract yourself from
other problems, worries or concerns?

Do you down-play how much you gamble
when talking with friends or family?

Is gambling the only solution you can
think of to pay debts?

Have you had to borrow money or sell any
belongings to enable you to gamble?

Are you tempted to keep gambling,
regardless of whether you've won or lost,
and just feel the need to have another go?

If you have honestly answered yes to one or more of these questions, it's likely that your gambling might have become a problem. Recognizing this is the first step towards getting help. It's important to take things one day at a time.

To help address this problem in its early stages, consider:

- Finding someone to talk with about it and support your plans, whether that's a friend or relative or a specialist counsellor or advisor

- Trying to stay away from places that might tempt you to gamble, but if that's too much in the first instance, set yourself some specific limits on the number of days or hours you'll gamble

- Limiting the amount of money you spend gambling, setting a limit and leaving cash or credit cards at home if you're going out to gamble

- Thinking about how you're managing your money so that it's not blown on gambling, making sure you pay your rent or mortgage and other costs of living first before you're tempted to gamble

There are numerous organizations and charities who can offer free support and advice to help cut down or stop gambling, including Gamcare which runs the National Gambling Helpline (0808 8020 133) and provides confidential information, advice and support for anyone affected by problem gambling in England, Scotland and Wales.[21] Gamblers Anonymous runs meetings around the world, offering advice and information, as well as access to their 12-step recovery programme.[22]

NURTURING YOUR MENTAL HEALTH FOLLOWING BEREAVEMENT

Reactions to loss and bereavement can vary greatly; there really is no right or wrong way to respond to this sad, troubling and often unexpected situation. The way you feel following the death of a loved one, friend, family member or colleague, whatever your reaction might be, is perfectly normal and doesn't mean that there's anything wrong with you.

Some common feelings you might experience include anger, denial and disbelief, fear, depression, guilt, numbness, mood swings, sadness, shock, lack of confidence and reliving memories. You may even experience a sense of guilt if you never expressed how you really felt about the person, or if there was a misunderstanding that was never cleared up before they passed away.

It is important to give yourself permission to feel the way you do rather than the way you think you should. Nonetheless, there are things you can do to help overcome the emotional pain being experienced.

- **Give yourself time to grieve:** It can take a long time, probably longer than you initially think, to adjust to a major bereavement.

- **It can help to talk:** Talking things through, sharing memories and expressing how feelings can help process your emotional reaction to the loss suffered.

- **It's also OK not to talk:** If you don't feel like talking, that is perfectly OK as well, but make sure that you talk to someone at some point to avoid becoming too isolated and withdrawn.

- **Take things slowly:** When recently bereaved, you will naturally feel anxious and worried and you might be struggling to concentrate. Be aware of the stress that you are under and take things slowly to avoid having an unnecessary accident or increasing your stress levels.

- **Don't feel guilty about moving on:** There will be a time when it is right to start rebuilding your life, so don't feel guilty when that happens. You're not being disloyal to the one who passed away.

- **Prepare yourself for the future:** There will be birthdays, anniversaries and other significant days that you will want to mark, especially during the first year after a bereavement. Think about how you can celebrate and commemorate these days, perhaps taking time off work or planning a special event with friends and family.

- **Keep keepsakes and memories around you:** Use photographs and other treasured possessions to keep the memories of your loved one alive. At some point you may be more able to celebrate their life, rather than dwelling on a visual memory of how they were when they passed away. Photos or videos of good times with them can help in this process.

- **Eat well, drink less and keep moving:** It is tempting to rely on alcohol or other drugs to try and numb the pain of bereavement, but in the longer term they can create other health problems, so it's best to avoid them or moderate your intake. Eating a balanced diet, getting some light exercise and taking plenty of rest will also help you to manage this difficult time.

Alongside the emotional pain of loss or bereavement, there are practical consequences associated with losing someone close, including housing and legal issues, childcare and support difficulties, as well as financial pressures. Arranging the funeral can create complications, especially if family members are dispersed or if there are tensions between people.

Talking with your doctor is a great starting point, especially if your distress is overwhelming. They may be able to recommend a counsellor who can help you to adjust to what has happened and help minimize the impact of your bereavement on your mental health.

LGBTQ+ AND MENTAL HEALTH

Although anyone can experience mental health difficulties, it's regrettable that LGBTQ+ (lesbian, gay, bisexual, trans, non-binary, queer or questioning) are more likely to develop a mental health problem.

In fact, more than 40% of LGBTQ+ people will experience a significant mental health problem, compared with about 25% of the general population.[23] Members of the LGBTQ+ community are also more likely to experience a range of mental health problems such as depression, suicidal thoughts, self-harm and alcohol and substance misuse.[24, 25, 26]

This state of affairs is likely in part a result of the stigma and discrimination that LGBTQ+ people face in their day-to-day lives. Sadly, one in six members of this community is expected to experience homophobic, biphobic or transphobic hate crime at some point in their lives, whether that's verbal abuse in the street or closer to home, or even a violent attack.[27]

And when it comes to the workplace, nearly three-quarters (74%) of LGBT+ people reported they had experienced mental health problems relating to work.[28] Added to this, 19% of LGBTQ+ employees have experienced verbal bullying from colleagues, customers or service users because of their sexual orientation in the last five years and 15% of lesbian, gay and bisexual employees have experienced verbal homophobic bullying from their colleagues in the last five years.[29]

Of course, there is more to us as individuals than our sexual orientation or gender identity and there are other cultural, socio-economic, demographic and age character-istics which influence how we feel about ourselves, as well as how others see us. But the prejudice and discrimination, including negative reactions or hostility from family mem-bers, strangers and even employers, means that too often LGBTQ+ people feel they cannot be open about their sex-ual orientation or gender which can, in turn, contribute to stress, tension and anxiety, as well as low self-esteem.

Alongside the barriers presented by prejudice and discrim-ination, there are other situations that can contribute to mental health problems for the LGBTQ+ community:

- **Coming out**
  Although for some, 'coming out' for the first time is an exciting and liberating experience, for others it's a huge challenge that threatens them with rejection or further harassment and isolation, resulting in negative feelings towards sexuality or gender identity. Coming out gradually, at least to one supportive person, can increase wellbeing, help manage the process, bolstering confidence and self-worth.

- **Substance abuse and misuse**
  LGBTQ+ people may be more likely to use drugs than heterosexual people. In fact, lesbian and bisexual women are more at risk of substance dependence than the rest of the population, with illegal drug use being four times higher than among heterosexual women.[30]

- **Accessing healthcare**
  LGBTQ+ people can experience more social isolation than the general population which can mean it's harder for them to get the support and treatment they need for physical and mental health issues. Aligned with this, there is also the danger that LGBTQ+ people, as well as those caring for them, may experience discrimination which creates a barrier to accessing healthcare services. A survey found that in gay and bisexual men who have accessed healthcare services, more than one third (34%) had a negative experience related to their sexual orientation, compared with half of lesbian and bisexual women.

The process of addressing mental health issues as a LGBTQ+ is similar to the approach that a heterosexual person might take, but the key is to get support from someone who understands your situation and context. Maybe it's a friend who's been there before, but if you decide to work with a professional counsellor, make sure you're comfortable with them and that they have a deep understanding of gender identity or sexual orientation contexts. It's not your job to educate them; they should be informed and educated to be able to help you from the outset.

With the right support, those diagnosed with mental health conditions can still enjoy a healthy, productive and happy life.

TRANSGENDER AND MENTAL HEALTH

Mental health and wellbeing are of particular importance for transgender individuals. The range of emotions and challenges experienced by transgender individuals can give rise to feelings of depression and anxiety and 40% of transgender adults have suicidal thoughts and attempts.[31]

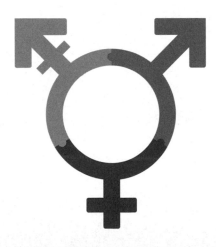

Whilst the range of issues that transgender individuals experience can massively impact their mental health, it is important to note that being a transgender doesn't mean other life issues won't impact their mental health and wellbeing. It's often hard to isolate these or seek help for other issues when your gender dysphoria – the underlying unease or dissatisfaction with your biological sex – is such a fundamental concern.

- **Gender dysphoria:** The uneasiness that you might feel with your biological sex can contribute to feelings of anxiety, depression and restlessness. It can also influence feelings of social anxiety and isolation if you feel under pressure to conform to what you believe to be social norms and expectations.

- **Decisions about transition:** Whether to transition or what level to transition to and how 'best' to transition are difficult decisions that require time and consideration. You might feel anxious and feel stressed about how your transition, at whatever stage you are at, you will be received and accepted by those closest to you, as well as strangers. You might also not wish to transition fully, instead identifying as 'gender queer' or 'third sex'. Equally, your decision to reveal your true self might be a very positive decision and one which, in fact, helps to nurture and improve your mental health.

- **Making your transition decision happen:** Even once you have decided to transition, your mental health may still be at risk as you come to terms with your new life. You might feel anxious and stressed about the impact of your decision on personal relationships or your colleagues and your employer. You might also be having surgeries and other medical treatments, which will impact how you feel, your resilience and emotional wellbeing.

It's important to remember that the process of transitioning will not be an immediate cure to any existing issues or mental health problems; you may still need to work through these in the same way as anyone else to ensure they are addressed and dealt with. Despite this, transitioning can give you a positive foundation on which to move forward.

"The thought of transitioning was daunting for me, it felt like a massive secret that was weighing me down. I struggled with depression and anxiety, as well as self-harm and I constantly felt nervous and uncomfortable. Now I've completed my transition, my mental health has drastically improved. Although it was a huge change for me, as well as my family, friends and work colleagues, it's been the best thing. I'm happier and more content and my mental health has completely improved."

POSITIVELY MANAGING YOUR OWN HEALTH AND WELLBEING

Ultimately it only takes one small change to start making a positive difference in your mental health, but this change has to be driven and managed by you. Here are some suggestions for how to better manage your mental health and wellbeing going forward.

- **Identify and build support networks:** Identify support networks that are available to you, find out how to take advantage of them and face up to the fact that it is OK to ask for help. Sometimes just being with people and enjoying their company is a great boost.

- **Be transparent:** Accept that it is OK to let others know when things are difficult. Everyone feels vulnerable at some point, so avoid getting trapped in a persona of someone who always copes.

- **Don't put all your eggs in one basket:** This includes not putting all your focus on work and neglecting your personal life and priorities.

- **Think about how you manage your time:** Take regular breaks for rest and relaxation when you're at work. Just because you may be working away from home or within a small team, don't be tempted to work 24 hours a day. This will only result in stress and burnout.

- **Establish realistic expectations for yourself:** It is important not to be a perfectionist, so give yourself a break and accept that mistakes will happen. How you learn and recover from these will shape your experience and your future.

- **Take care of yourself:** Do something positive to look after yourself, such as eating well, exercising, getting enough sleep and watching your alcohol intake. Make self-care an essential part of your daily routine.

- **Get enough rest:** Are you going home at a reasonable time? Are you taking all your holiday allocation? Are you looking at your work emails at home, just before going to bed or during the middle of the night when you can't sleep? Work-life balance is important and you need to ensure that you're creating quality rest time outside of work.

- **Deal with problems effectively:** Changing your perception of a problem may help find the solution. For example, think about what you can change about a situation or the way others perceive it, or talk through strategies for handling difficult problems with someone you trust.

- **Communicate assertively:** Try and find a balance between not bottling up feelings and not over-reacting. Try to communicate clearly, in a way that's respectful of yourself and others, and be comfortable saying 'no' when you need to.

- **Remain calm under pressure:** Think about what you can realistically do to change a situation. If there is nothing you can do about it, step back, remain calm and avoid making a rushed response. Sometimes something as simple as counting to ten gives a greater sense of perspective and helps avoid a knee-jerk reaction.

- **Get some perspective:** You can render smaller irritations irrelevant if you compare them with larger and more complex issues and situations. As the saying goes: 'Don't sweat the small stuff'. It's good to remember this from time to time.

- **Create positive experiences:** Do something to incorporate positive experiences into your daily life and routine. It's a good exercise to think what your ideal day would include, and then think about what you could do to make this dream a reality. What do you need to change in order to make this happen?

PART 3

UNDER-
STANDING
SPECIFIC
MENTAL
HEALTH
CONDITIONS

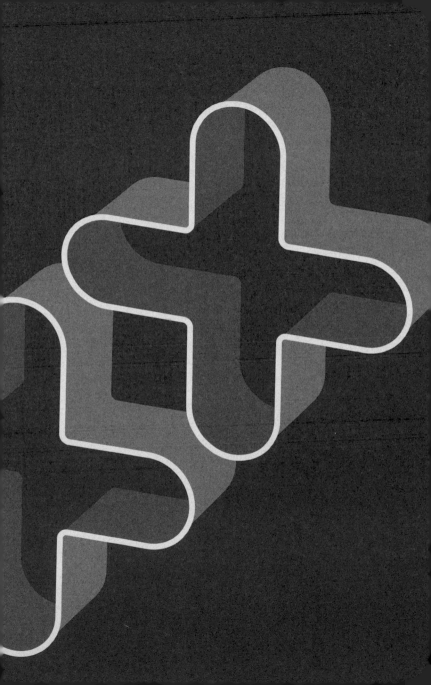

HOW STRESS AND PRESSURE AFFECT MENTAL HEALTH

It's all too common to hear a friend, colleague or person in the street declaring that they feel 'stressed'. And although we use the term a lot, it can be hard to define exactly what it means.

It is probably not helpful to know that 'stress' is not in itself a medical term. There isn't a medical definition of 'stress', and there continues to be debate about whether stress is the cause of problems you're experiencing, or the result of them.

The UK's health and safety regulator has helpfully defined stress as the "adverse reaction people have to excessive pressures or other types of demand placed on them".[32] Essentially, it is a set of reactions and responses that we each have to the day-to-day pressures we experience. In the rest of this chapter we will refer to 'stress' as meaning excessive pressure.

There are a lot of useful resources and information relating to stress on their website – take a look.

But whether stress is a mental health problem really depends on the individual.

Everyone reacts differently to pressure and, like it or not, it is a normal part of life that isn't going to go away. One person might find it a strong source of motivation and be energized by stress, whereas another might be overwhelmed by it and struggle to cope under the pressure. An individual's response to it can also depend on what else is going on in their personal or work life.

Stress can in fact cause mental health problems, leading to anxiety and depression, for example, or making these and other mental health conditions worse. In turn, mental health problems can increase stress, because of the struggles in coping with day-to-day symptoms and treatments.

If you think you might be suffering from stress, there are some physical and emotional symptoms that you might be able to identify. These include difficulty sleeping, tearfulness, exhaustion, headaches, neck or back pain, obsessive behaviour, heart palpitations, panic attacks, feelings of pointlessness or futility, struggling to focus or concentrate, or eating, smoking or drinking more than you normally would.

And in the workplace, you might find yourself having more conflict with colleagues, struggling with the pressures of work, finding reasons to take more time off or finding it difficult to get to work on time. You might also notice a decline in your performance and that you're delivering less work than usual.

"Whenever I feel stressed and under pressure, I try to remove myself from that situation for about five to ten minutes. I take time out to breathe and clear my mind and thought process. This helps me a lot to calm down and then I can go back into the situation without pressure and can think of a situation more clearly."

MINIMIZING THE IMPACT OF STRESS

If you are feeling stressed, it is highly likely that you need to take notice – and take action – to change things. Fortunately, there are positive steps for responding to and minimizing the impact of stress.

- **Keep on top of your physical and emotional health**
  Lifestyle is intrinsically linked to mental and physical health and so a healthy lifestyle will help you to stay alert and cope, should things become stressful. This means paying attention to eating healthily, keeping fit, making time to relax, not smoking and watching your alcohol intake.

  ▸ Regular exercise will increase your capacity to cope with stress. It releases those 'feel good hormones', endorphins, and helps give a sense of perspective and 'time out' if pressure starts to increase. Of course, if you haven't been keeping yourself moving recently, it is always best to visit your doctor for a check-up before launching into an exercise programme.

▸ Most of us are familiar with the idea of eating at least five portions of fruit and vegetables, as well as drinking up to two litres of water, every day. It is equally important to eat foods rich in starches and fibre, choose fish or lean cuts of meat and poultry, and to avoid too much salty or sugary food. All of this will help manage stress levels and maintain good physical health.

▸ Moderate alcohol consumption isn't a bad thing, but at stressful times there is a danger of becoming dependent on alcohol to help manage, rather than address the factors that are causing it. The same can be said of smoking. Cutting down or cutting out both of these temptations will have a positive effect on your physical and mental health.

- **Look at how organized you really are**
A major factor that leads to high stress levels is feeling a lack of control, whether that's at home, with family life or at work. But introducing a few simple rules for managing day-to-day responsibilities can make a massive difference.

  ▸ **Use one method to organize your day and your life:** Whether it's a paper diary, an electronic desktop diary or an app, keeping everything well ordered, in one place, will reduce the chances of double-booking and missing appointments. It will also help identify upcoming busy and potentially stressful times, giving you the chance to prepare and make alternative arrangements before it is too late.

- **Take a break at every opportunity:** This works on a range of levels, but each will help to minimize feelings of stress:

  » Rather than booking back-to-back appointments or work tasks, give yourself some breathing space between each one to gather thoughts, sort actions from your previous appointment or just grab a breather.

  » Also, unless you've mastered time travel, remember to block out sufficient travel time between appointments, whether they're across town or with a colleague on a different floor of your building.

  » The same is true for lunch breaks. In fact, just giving yourself permission to have a lunch break could be a major step forward!

  » Schedule some 'desk' or 'thinking' time that will help get your administration done or prepare an important piece of work. Make sure to block the time out in your diary so other people don't encroach on it.

  » Make note of all leisure or personal commitments in your work diary, giving them the same importance as other items in your schedule.

- **Be realistic about how long a task will take:** It is tempting to agree to ambitious schedules only to discover later that they are just impossible to deliver on. Try giving yourself too much time to complete something rather than creating pressure to meet an unrealistic deadline.

▸ **Keep communicating, especially if things aren't going to plan:** If someone isn't following the 'rules' to book appointments or tasks in your diary, and that is putting you under pressure, make sure to let them know and explain how to better manage it all. Politely, of course!

If you are struggling to deliver a task or project on time, talk to your customer or the project team about it. Sharing the problem and finding a solution that works for everyone is the best way to reduce such stresses.

• **Stop ... and relax!**
The thought of relaxing when feeling stressed might seem impossible but developing the ability to unwind after you've had a bad day will reduce stress levels and help give you a positive outlook moving forward.

When stressed, upset or nervous, muscles in your body naturally tighten. You might feel hot, sweaty or on edge, your heart may be racing and your breathing could seem faster and shallower than usual. By finding a relaxation technique that works for you at stressful times, you can better manage these situations.

▸ Learning how to control your breathing is an important part of being able to relax effectively. You can do this by following the simple instructions below, but don't forget to consult your doctor before undertaking a new exercise regime, or if this technique causes you any discomfort.

» Lay on the floor, placing one hand on your abdomen (or stomach) and the other on your upper chest. Relax like this for a few minutes and get used to your breathing. Feel the rise and fall of the breathing with your hands.

» Then, inhale slowly and deeply and try to push out the lower hand by breathing in deep into your stomach. Continue to inhale and exhale deeply and try to keep your rib cage and upper hand still – so your lower hand on your stomach is pushed up and down but the upper hand on your chest is not.

» Exhale through your mouth, making a quiet 'whooshing' noise as you blow out gently.

» Continue to breathe in and out slowly.

Repeat this daily for about ten minutes for the greatest benefit. With practice, you should be able to slow your breathing down to about four or five breaths per minute.

Another exercise you can try, either sitting or lying down, is to breathe in through your nose, counting up to five, and then gradually letting your breath come out through your mouth, counting up to eight as you breathe out. Repeat this, trying to make sure the length of your 'out' breath is double that of the breath you take in.

Have you tried mindfulness?

Mindfulness is a process to relax the body and remove negative thoughts through a deepened state of relaxation. It's about becoming mindful of the 'here and now' and by focusing – being mindful – of the moment, you can better understand and appreciate the impact that negative thoughts can have on you and your health. Too often in our busy lives, we jump from one thing to another and are distracted from what's happening. So we forget to focus on the moment that we're in.

The key to mindfulness is finding a physical space where you feel comfortable and can relax, closing the eyes and focusing on what needs to be improved or changed. It's about visualizing how to get there and what the result would look like. If you find your mind wandering away from your attempts to be mindful, bring your focus back to your breathing and the space you've found for yourself.

Guided imagery is a great way to adopt mindfulness as it uses similar meditation techniques but makes use of an image or story to guide your thinking. There are loads of resources online that offer guided imagery for a range of situations and circumstances, such as reducing stress, anxiety and depression, as well as helping you to relax. (See positivepsychologyprogram.com/interactive-guided-imagery-therapy).

As with mindfulness, guided imagery should be used in a quiet place where you can focus on yourself, your thoughts and your breathing. And importantly, in the case of both these techniques, it's a case of the more you do it, the bigger the benefits you can reap as it becomes second nature to help yourself relax and reduce stress and anxiety.

- **Change the way you think**
  A positive mental attitude will definitely help you cope when feeling stressed or under pressure. We have all been guilty of thinking irrationally about a person or a situation, and that does nothing to solve the problem we believe we're experiencing.

  ▸ You have an 'all or nothing' mindset, and if something falls slightly short of perfection or success, you consider it a total failure.

  ▸ You see a single negative event or experience as a constant pattern of defeat, and even though it might have only happened once, you use words like 'always' or 'never' to describe what has happened.

  ▸ You pick out one negative detail and dwell on it, obscuring everything else that may be positive about a situation.

  ▸ You jump to conclusions, interpreting things as negative even when there are no facts to back up your thinking.

  The best way to stop thinking in this negative way is to try and become aware that you are doing this – recognizing it is the first step. Try to use more positive vocabulary and take a step back from a situation to weigh up all the evidence before you reach any conclusions or make decisions.

- **Don't be afraid to put yourself first**
  Being aware of the importance of speaking up for yourself, saying 'no' and putting yourself or your interests first can help avoid feeling that you have no control or choice over something.

  Being assertive in this way means respecting yourself – this is who you are and this is what you do – and taking responsibility for how you feel, what you think and the actions you take. Here, it is important to let yourself make mistakes, recognizing that these will happen and that you can learn from them.

  To help put your interests and feelings first, you could adopt a number of tactics:

  ▸ Ask for time to think something over; don't be made to rush into a decision.

  ▸ Ask for what you need, rather than hoping that someone else will already know this and take action on your behalf.

  ▸ Distinguish between having a responsibility towards other people, but not being responsible for other people. These are two very different things.

It is easy to delay seeking help when you're feeling stressed, or to wait before taking positive action to make a change. Perhaps you just hope that things will change naturally, or you don't want to ask for help because you think that would be an admission of failure.

Unfortunately, these matters generally won't resolve themselves.

If you're struggling to manage alone, it is probably time to ask for professional help and guidance, whether that is from your doctor, your manager or services such as your company's EAP or Occupational Health service. All of these are confidential, and you are in control of what happens, but nothing can change until you recognize that you need help and are willing to accept it.

BURNOUT

When your stress becomes unmanageable and continues for a prolonged period, there is a danger that it can develop into what is commonly known as 'burnout'. This is not a clinical term, but an informal description of how mentally and emotionally run down and depleted you can end up feeling over time.

Burnout is a gradual process and it builds on many of the signs and symptoms of stress, creating a sense of mental, physical and emotional exhaustion that leaves you feeling helpless, disillusioned and struggling to gather the energy to do the simplest tasks.

When you reach burnout, you really are at rock bottom: even the smallest problem feels impossible to tackle, you are constantly unhappy, and the future looks bleak. Your energy levels will be low and the way you're feeling will be having a very negative impact on your family, your physical and mental health and your work. You've basically run out of resources to cope.

It is important to recognize that whilst burnout can be the result of constant and unrelenting stress, it is not the same as stress. Stress can be the result of many factors, including too many demands, requirements or pressures in your work or home life. People who are under stress believe they will get better once they get on top of these things.

In contrast, burnout is about feeling empty and seriously lacking motivation. People suffering from burnout just can't see any hope or a way that their situation can change. They have no drive or energy to try and make things different, even if they wanted to.

Burnout can be caused by a number of factors specific to an individual and the type of roles and responsibilities they have in their life.

- At work you might feel like you have little or no control over what you are being asked to do, you might be frustrated that you're getting no recognition or reward for what you're doing, and you might be anxious that you're not clear about what is expected of you or that too many demands are being placed on your time. It is also possible that you might be in a very repetitive, monotonous job or that your workplace is a particularly chaotic, high-pressure environment.

- Your lifestyle might contribute to burnout, with too much time spent at work making it difficult to find enough time to relax. Or you might have taken on too many responsibilities with insufficient help or support from other people. You might also be missing close relationships or not getting enough sleep.

- You may be a perfectionist and nothing you do or attempt to do is good enough. Alternatively, you might have a pessimistic view of the world and your place in it. You might also want to be in control and find it hard to delegate even straightforward tasks, instead insisting on taking everything on yourself.

Some of the symptoms of burnout can be very subtle, but as they get worse the signs will intensify as your body absorbs the stress. That is why it is particularly important to 'listen' to your body and get some help before things get too bad. Taking action at the earliest opportunity will prevent a full-blown breakdown.

Here are some questions to consider if you think you might be on the road to burnout:

- Do you feel tired and physically 'drained' all of the time?
- Are you suffering from frequent headaches or muscular pain?
- Have you spotted a change in your appetite or sleeping habits?
- Are you getting sick a lot, catching every bug and cold that goes around?
- Have you lost motivation to do even the simplest tasks?
- Are you becoming increasingly cynical and negative about things?
- Does every day feel like a bad day?
- Do you opt to call in sick rather than tackle what needs to be done?
- Have you begun to feel helpless, trapped or alone?
- Have you lost a sense of satisfaction with work, and life in general?
- Does it take much longer to get things done, whether at home or work?
- Do you pull away and isolate yourself from friends and family?

- Do you get snappy and take your frustrations out on others?
- Have you turned to food, alcohol, cigarettes or drugs to help you cope with things?
- Do you feel that nothing you do makes a difference or is appreciated?

If you answer yes to some or all of these questions, there is a chance that you may have reached burnout. Certainly, if you are feeling this way, it is time to give yourself a break and ask for some help from your GP or a health professional. There is also a chance that you might be experiencing the symptoms of a clinical condition, such as anxiety, depression or both, so there really is no time like the present to seek help.

"When I experienced burnout, it was the support from my manager that made the biggest difference to my recovery. At first, I found it really difficult to ask for help but when I did, I received such a positive and supportive reaction. My manager asked how she could support me and if I needed to take time out to recuperate, but it was the ongoing conversations and knowing she was there and cared that made the biggest difference. When you're in the spiral of burnout it's really hard to see out of it and every little thing feels like a massive issue at the time. Talking to my manager helped to take the little things away and to talk constructively about the big things. Don't be afraid of asking for help, my biggest regret was not talking to my manager sooner."

Don't be
afraid of asking
for help.

CAN YOU OVERCOME BURNOUT?

When suffering with burnout, reaching out to others is one of the most effective ways of dealing with how you're feeling. Just finding someone who can listen, who won't judge or be easily distracted from what you're saying, is a great first step in relieving some of the pressure you are under.

If you are ready to deal with burnout, here are some more tips:

- **Develop the positive relationships in your life**
  - ▸ Invest time in those closest to you. Try your best to put how you are feeling to one side and just spend time together, focusing on the moment rather than what will happen next.

  - ▸ Try to engage with the people you work with, just having a chat while you're making a cup of tea or arranging social events after work. This will help put work and what's being asked of you into perspective, and provide a sounding board when things get tough.

▸ Avoid people who are always negative, especially if they are continually complaining about things. They will only bring you down, so it's best to steer clear!

▸ Team up with people who share similar interests, whether it's a sports club, a social club or a religious group. These will give you the chance to talk and interact with people who have the same interests. It's a great way to get out the house and expand your social circle.

- **Re-think and re-frame how you're feeling**
  ▸ For most, it is just not possible or practical to quit a job we're not happy with and find a new one. So instead, reflect on what you are doing and try to find some value in it. Think about how your work might be helping others or focus on the parts that you do enjoy, even if it's simply the banter with co-workers during a tea break.

  ▸ If you are feeling frustrated and demotivated by your work, can you find a few hours to do some volunteer work every week? This has the potential to add meaning and satisfaction to your life, hopefully without impacting your paid job too heavily.

- **Think about what and who you can change at work**
  ▸ Who are your friends at work? Having friendships at work can reduce the feelings of monotony, and laughing and joking with friends during the workday can reduce stress and keep you going when you're feeling down.

But do consider whether the jokes and banter in the workplace are helpful. Are they actually a smoke-screen that serves to avoid talking about the real issues that are affecting not just you but also your associates at work?

▸ Can you take some time off? A great way to address burnout is to take time away from work and remove yourself completely from what may be contributing to how you feel.

- **Re-evaluate and re-define your priorities**
  ▸ Being burned out is a sign that something isn't quite right in your life, so take the hint and reflect on your goals and dreams. Have you drifted away from something that's truly important to you and makes you happy? What can you do to reconnect with that person, place or thing?

  ▸ Be prepared to say no, especially when people are put-ting unnecessary and unacceptable demands on your time. The first time is the hardest – after you've said 'no' once and freed yourself up, it will be much easier going forward.

  ▸ Set yourself free from technology by making time every day to completely disconnect from your phone, tablet, PC and/or Kindle, even your personal fitness tracker. It is OK to be unavailable and unmonitored, so enjoy the freedom and accept the peace of feeling unconnected.

- **Exercise, rest and refuel**
  - ▸ Although it is probably the last thing you feel like doing when you're burned out, exercise is a powerful mood booster. Just 30 minutes' exercise every day – or even three lots of 30 minutes a week – can improve your mood.

  - ▸ Make time to relax during the day, even for a few minutes. Sit quietly, close your eyes and focus on your breathing. Getting a good quality night's sleep will also help to keep you focused and combat the symptoms of burnout.

  - ▸ Your diet has a massive impact on how you're feeling and the energy levels you're able to tap into. Try to minimize your intake of sugary foods, as well as those with high levels of refined carbohydrates, trans-fats and preservatives. Cutting down on caffeine and drinking alcohol in moderation will also help reduce your feelings of anxiety.

Overcoming burnout isn't an easy thing to do, but it's not impossible. By taking the first step of just talking with someone else, you can start to regain control of your feelings and your outlook until you're firmly on the road to recovery.

DEALING WITH TRAUMA

Trauma is defined by the Oxford English Dictionary as 'a powerful shock that may have long lasting effects' and it can relate to a wide range of situations and circumstances that present a real or perceived threat or danger to us as individuals.

Between 7% and 14% of people will experience a traumatic event at some point in their lives.[33] Furthermore, about 10% of these people will develop trauma-related illnesses and are likely to have longer-term symptoms that would benefit from professional help and intervention.

Traumatic events might include an accident, natural disaster, fire, car crash, violent attack, an act or threat of terrorism, or some other crime-related violence or threat.

The response to these events depends on a number of factors, including previous exposure to trauma, how it was managed and the support networks available. Our personality, emotional resilience and life experiences, as well as our level of self-awareness and ability to express feelings, will dictate how we react and recover.

In the immediate aftermath of a traumatic event we are likely to be in shock and distressed. Our heart will probably beat faster, we may feel sick and our mouth will be dry. Talking coherently might be difficult and our thoughts will be jumbled. Whilst the way we feel will be disturbing, it is a natural reaction to our 'fight or flight' instinct and not a sign of mental illness.

In the longer term, physical and emotional responses to trauma can be more wide-ranging and may include:

- Intrusive or unwelcome thoughts
- Difficulty concentrating
- Confusion and disorientation
- Amnesia or memory loss
- Nervousness and anxiety
- Withdrawal from people and situations
- Sadness, depression and feelings of vulnerability
- Difficulty relating to other people
- Anger and irritability
- Poor sleep and nightmares
- Increased or loss of appetite
- Increased alcohol or drug intake
- Hyper-vigilance and alertness
- Replaying events and obsessing over different outcomes

Of course, most people who experience a traumatic event will gradually recover within the first few weeks. And whilst this recovery is unlikely to involve completely forgetting the incident, over time, troubling memories and anxiety will fade.

However, if these symptoms continue for some time, they're likely to start affecting your mental health. It is at this stage that professional help would definitely be beneficial.

Your mental health will also benefit from calm and supportive friends and family who are able to help you process what has happened and help you get back on track to a 'normal' life.

+ TREATMENTS FOR TRAUMA

The two main recommended treatments are Trauma Focused Cognitive Behavioural Therapy (TF-CBT) and Eye Movement Desensitisation and Reprocessing (EMDR), although before these treatments are implemented, healthcare practitioners may adopt a 'watchful waiting' approach which monitors how an individual's symptoms and feelings are changing.[34]

- **Trauma Focused Cognitive Behavioural Therapy:** This is a form of talking treatment with a trained, professional therapist during eight to 12 weekly sessions of up to 90 minutes each. TF-CBT helps deal with overwhelming problems in a positive way by breaking them down into smaller elements. As part of this, the therapist helps to change these negative thought patterns into practical ways to improve the individual's state of mind. And importantly, it focuses on the traumatic experiences in order to give the patient some relief from any negative self-critical beliefs that may have crept in.

- **Eye Movement Desensitisation and Reprocessing:** This is a relatively new treatment that can help minimize some of the symptoms of Post-traumatic stress disorder (PTSD) and trauma, such as becoming easily startled. The treatment involves briefly reliving traumatic experiences while the therapist directs eye movements (or they can tap the patient or get them to watch a light move from side to side – whichever method used, these stimulate the brain bilaterally). There is strong evidence that this treatment will help process the emotional elements of the traumatic experiences and desensitize them, thereby helping the individual to cope with them more effectively. (For more information go to www.emdrassociation.org.uk)

SUPPORTING YOUR MENTAL HEALTH IN THE AFTERMATH OF TRAUMA

Sometimes people who have experienced a traumatic event go on to develop Post-Traumatic Stress Disorder (PTSD). If you are suffering from this condition, you will certainly require professional help to recover.

Fortunately, there are positive actions that support mental health in the aftermath of a traumatic event:

- **Accept that things take time:** It is important to acknowledge that it will take time to recover from the experience, but if you're still dealing with the effects of the incident after one month, seek medical help.

- **Keep people close to you:** In the wake of a traumatic incident, it's tempting to keep to yourself and withdraw from social situations, but it is important to stay connected and keep people, especially those that you can open up to, close to you.

- **Maintain your routines:** Keeping to a regular routine will help to get you back on track. This includes sleep times, meal times and trying to get back to work.

- **Try and stay at work:** Work gives you the opportunity to stay connected with other people, in this case your colleagues. If the trauma happened at work, access the support services within your organization to help you recover.

- **Stay on track:** Although it can be tempting to drink excessive alcohol or turn to recreational drugs to help numb the memories in the aftermath of a traumatic incident, these can actually intensify your symptoms and 'self-medicating' with them should be avoided.

- **Recognize that what you are feeling is perfectly normal:** Regardless of how you are feeling in the aftermath of a trauma – whether your feelings and emotions are more intense and unpredictable than usual, or if you don't feel different at all – this is perfectly normal. We all react differently and need different types of support, information and reassurance to help overcome trauma.

- **Take time to relax and refresh:** Keeping up with hobbies and pastimes will assist recovery, as will finding the time to relax and unwind. This will allow your mind and body to recover from the experience they've been through.

Ultimately, it is important to remember that trauma can be a life-changing experience, and whilst it can be meaningful and significant at the time, most people do recover. It is important to be patient with yourself.

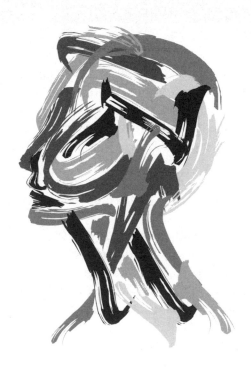

UNDERSTANDING ANXIETY

It is perfectly natural to feel anxious, apprehensive or worried from time to time. Feeling like this is a normal reaction to a temporarily stressful situation like starting a new job, delivering a presentation, taking a test or meeting someone new, especially if it is an important meeting.

Most of the time, our feelings of concern subside as soon as the situation is over and we become more relaxed.

However, there are times when this isn't the case and feelings of anxiety stay for a long period of time, causing overwhelm and panic. As a result, mental health will suffer, and over time feelings like this can affect interactions with others, performance and attendance at work, sleep patterns and day-to-day routines. There is also a danger when anxiety becomes overwhelming and because it can't be controlled these feelings can lead to depression.

!¡!

Anxiety levels are one of the indicators for overall personal wellbeing alongside how satisfied you're feeling with your life, the extent you feel things in your life are worthwhile and how happy you feel. According to the Office of National Statistics, average anxiety levels for the UK reached a three-year low in 2018, but this still amounts to 10.3 million people continuing to report high anxiety scores.[35]

The symptoms of anxiety will vary from person to person and at a psychological level might include fear, being on edge, irritability, difficulty concentrating and relaxing, feeling weepy and dependent, and seeking reassurance from others.

Physically, the muscular tension of feeling this way can cause headaches and increased blood pressure. Added to this, more rapid breathing can cause light-headedness or pins and needles, and even nausea. Longer term, anxiety can weaken the immune system and make people more susceptible to infections. Higher blood pressure can increase the risks of having a stroke, heart and kidney problems, as well as depression.

So, learning to recognize and control anxiety is an important step towards good mental and physical health and wellbeing. Fortunately, though, there are a number of ways that you can help yourself.

- It is imperative to confront anxiety and how it makes you feel. Keep reminding yourself how much better you will feel when feelings of apprehension are reduced to a more manageable level

- Use breathing and relaxation techniques to proactively manage some of the symptoms of anxiety. Alternatively, listening to relaxing music, taking up disciplines such as yoga or meditation, or simply taking the time to enjoy a hot bath can help break the cycle

- Looking after yourself physically is also important. Get some exercise and release some endorphins to improve your mood. But also try to avoid things like caffeine, cigarettes and alcohol, as they can intensify your feelings of anxiety. Getting good quality rest and sleep – and eating a good, balanced diet topped up with plenty of water – will also improve your feelings

- Talking through what makes you feel anxious will help to put your thoughts and feelings into context; it really does help to confide in a friend or family member, your doctor or a counsellor. Also remember that your employer may have invested in an EAP that can offer independent, confidential support and information at any hour of the day or night

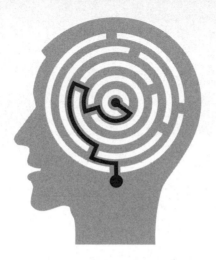

"I've been able to put a stop to feelings of anxiety by knowing that it is a human reaction and know that it is never as bad as it first appears. Taking perspective and also trying to teach yourself to enjoy the experience or to focus on how you will feel when you come through the other side will all help."

PUTTING A STOP TO FEELINGS OF ANXIETY

Changing the way you think is one of the most important things you can do to stop anxiety.

- When you start to get anxious, just stop what you're doing. Can you identify the feelings and patterns of thinking that made you feel this way? What is going on around you that could have contributed to this feeling?

- Can you see where the anxiety-related thoughts are originating? Perhaps you are looking at something out of perspective. Is there another way to look at or interpret the situation?

- Do you assume the worst and just expect to fail? How would you feel if you anticipated the best, or at least a somewhat better outcome?

- How do you regard the future? Can you look forward positively, or do you look at the past and dwell on events that simply can't be changed?

- Are you becoming overly self-critical? Feeling anxious can encourage you to be critical of yourself and others, so try to take a step back and look at the positives

- Do you tend to blame yourself when things go wrong? How can you challenge yourself to re-think what has happened and why?

- Who else might have some responsibility for the outcome of a situation, and if you were giving advice to them, how might you help them to feel better about the outcome and themselves?

Asking yourself these questions and trying some of the strategies presented here is a great place to start if you're experiencing anxiety and want to do something about it. But if these don't work for you, it is worth considering the professional medical support that is available via your doctor, EAP or a professional counsellor.

RECOGNIZING THE SIGNS OF DEPRESSION

Everyone feels sad or down at different points life, and feeling this way is the body's natural reaction to a loss or change or even a physical medical condition. But if these feelings are persistent or occur regularly, there is a chance that they're highlighting the onset of depression.

The term depression covers a broad range of symptoms that can impact an individual's physical and mental health and wellbeing. Milder depression – lots of us would just call it 'the blues' – can make normal, day-to-day tasks a real challenge. For instance, this can mean feeling indifferent towards others and tasks, struggling to concentrate and finding it hard to make decisions.

When these feelings devolve into utter desperation or hopelessness, it is likely that the depression is severe or acute and there is a danger that thoughts of self-harm or suicide could accompany them.

Depression can affect people differently and at different times in their life. Some of the more common symptoms of depression include:

- Low self-esteem or self-worth
- Loss of sex drive
- Pessimistic view of life and the future
- Being unusually irritable
- Reduced energy levels and activity
- Feeling hopeless or helpless with strong negative thoughts
- Crying, or being unable to cry
- Self-harm or suicidal thoughts

Depression can be triggered by many things, from bereavement, bullying, loneliness and isolation, to the loss of a job or a series of challenges and setbacks in life. It can also accompany physical illness and can be intensified by increased alcohol intake, recreational drugs, poor diet and little or no exercise.

Your doctor is a great first point of contact if you think you are suffering from depression. They can offer appropriate treatment, which could include anti-depressants and/or counselling. Your employer might also have set up an EAP or have an in-house counselling or occupational health service, which are great ways of getting some fast-track professional help.

TIPS FOR OVERCOMING DEPRESSION

Alongside the professional help that is available for depression, there are also things you can do to help yourself:

- **Establish a routine:** A routine can help provide structure and framework to your life, especially if you're feeling so unwell that you are not at work. You might be surprised to know that being at work can really help with these feelings because it automatically gives a structure and routine and can help distract you from the negative thoughts.

- **Keep moving and keep eating:** Staying fit and healthy and getting regular exercise will release endorphins to boost positive mood, and when combined with a well-balanced diet, exercise can prevent you from feeling sluggish and lethargic.

- **Watch what you're drinking:** Alcohol is a depressant, which means it slows down the functions of the central nervous system and can further lower your mood, especially the morning after! Whilst it might be tempting to 'drown your sorrows', the benefits of this are short-lived and could lead to even greater feelings of depression.

- **Seek out a self-help group:** Groups like this work on the premise that meeting, talking and interacting with people who are experiencing similar feelings can help break down the sense of isolation and introduce new coping methods and strategies. It is also reassuring, and probably surprising, to realize that many other people, including well-known personalities and celebrities, struggle with depression. We're seeing more and more of them going on record to declare this as a way of encouraging others to talk.

- **Don't dismiss the benefits of medication:** Antidepressants work by balancing the chemicals in your brain called neurotransmitters, the ones that affect mood and emotions. This medicine can help to improve your mood, help you sleep more and help you to manage your appetite and concentration whilst you're getting yourself back on track. You can talk with your doctor about this, but it is something to consider if you're struggling with the symptoms of depression.

DEVELOPING A DEEPER UNDERSTANDING OF SUICIDE

Suicide isn't something that we really talk about much as a society, which is a concern because it is believed that one person in every 15 has made a suicide attempt at some point in their life.[36] In fact, more people die from suicide than from traffic accidents, according to the UK's Samaritans charity group.[37]

!¡!

Almost 5,000 people in England took their own life in 2015. Suicide is now the main cause of death for men under 50. Although women are less likely to die by suicide than men, the rate of female suicide is the highest in more than a decade.[38]

Suicide can be triggered by many different things, such as a long-term health condition or feelings of depression, hopelessness and despair associated with acute mental health problems. In the moment when you are suffering in this way, suicide might feel like the only option available to you, but there are other ways to regain control and achieve a positive outlook on life.

If you are having suicidal thoughts, it's important to talk with someone as soon as possible, maybe a close friend or a relative, or perhaps a health professional or your doctor. There are lots of organizations you can talk with anonymously and in confidence and who are there for you any time of the day.

If you are struggling to cope and have suicidal thoughts, please remember that there is help out there.

- When you feel able to seek support from a health professional, be honest and say exactly how you feel. They won't be shocked by what you are saying and, by being straight with them, you enable them to give you the treatment and, if necessary, the medication that you need

- If you're not clear about the treatment or medication they're prescribing, make sure you ask for more information and clarification. Follow the doctor's or counsellor's instructions; they've successfully helped lots of people before, so they're really well placed to help you too

- Don't be embarrassed or ashamed about how you're feeling. Mental health issues affect so many of us and there are lots of support systems, treatments and help to manage how you're feeling

Additionally, if you think someone close to you is suicidal, it is really important to act on your concerns.

- If you think it is appropriate, ask them if you can help

- Listen to them, without judgement or interruption

- Discuss your concerns or options in confidence with someone who can help, such as a professional who is expert in mental health

- If there is an immediate threat of suicide or serious self-harm, encourage the person to go to their local hospital's Accident & Emergency department. Alternatively, call for emergency medical help

Where you think that a person might be at risk of committing suicide, it is always better to overreact than wish later on that you had taken a particular course of action.

Many people can be affected by suicide, especially the family, friends and co-workers of the person who has taken this final step. Here, your emotional reaction to bereavement following a suicide can often be more intense, complicated and prolonged than if death was by natural causes. It will likely consist of a range of feelings, including:

- **Shock:** Finding it hard to accept what has happened or the way it did.

- **Confusion:** Finding it difficult to reconcile or understand what led to such a final act.

- **Despair and sadness:** A sense of hopelessness and intense sadness that has the potential to lead to depression.

- **Anger:** Directing anger towards the deceased, as inappropriate as this might feel, or their family or friends.

- **Blame:** Feeling that you or those close to the deceased may have missed clues, and blaming yourself or others for not preventing the suicide.

- **Grief:** These feelings depend on the individual, their relationship with the deceased and their previous experiences of bereavement, loss and suicide.

- **Guilt:** A persistent feeling that something might have helped the deceased, reflecting on last conversations and interactions and searching for clues about how they were feeling.

Each response to suicide is unique; some people may withdraw and find it hard to talk about what has happened, or prefer to deny what happened or how they're feeling. Other people may need to talk about their experiences. Whichever is best for those concerned, it is important that you do what feels right for you and, where possible, keep talking and ask for support and guidance as soon as you can.

PART 4

MENTAL HEALTH, TRANSITION AND TIMES OF CHANGE

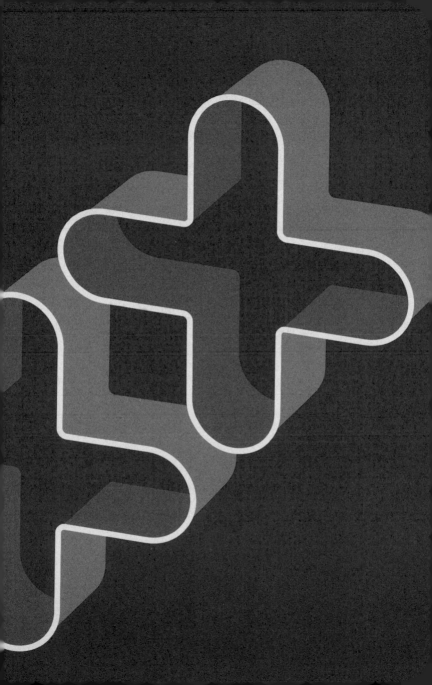

CHANGE AND MENTAL HEALTH

Change is inevitable, whether we proactively make it happen or it arrives unexpectedly. We can regard it as an opportunity or a challenge: our perception of it very much depends on us as individuals and our mental health. Because change is a part of life, it's something we need to learn to live and cope with.

Sometimes change can feel threatening, forcing us to face unknown situations. If we fear it, when it happens it is likely that change will worry or upset us and can negatively impact our mental health.

If we regard change as offering us a new and different set of options, it is likely that we will perceive it as exciting, allowing us to accept the change and believe that the choices it presents are within our control.

So by learning to accept and prepare for change, we can reduce the impact it has on us and our mental health. And, believe it or not, the ways to manage the response to change are relatively straightforward. Whilst most situations present their own unique challenges, there are some general 'rules'.

- **Think positively about the change you're facing**
  When it comes to change, most people have a huge fear of the unknown and this fear breeds worry and anxiety. It is easy to be negative about change, but by retaining an open and positive outlook and focusing on the elements that can be controlled, it can be made a more positive experience.

- **Take a step back from change**
  When going through a process or a period of change, it can feel all-consuming. You can get a better sense of perspective about what is happening by taking some time out, disengaging from what is going on, and allowing yourself to come back to things with a clean slate and a fresh perspective.

- **Be prepared to talk things through**
  When feeling anxious or concerned about change and the impact it might have on you and your life, it is always best to try and talk things through with a friend, family member or a health professional. Even though you might not reach a solution, just the process of talking can help to clarify your thoughts, identify further questions you want to ask or information to source and begin to define your response to the change and the challenges it presents.

- **Don't be afraid to get involved in change**
  Although it is tempting to avoid change, if you have the opportunity to get actively involved in it and express your opinion, it is more likely that you will feel comfortable with the changes that are being proposed. Having the chance to express your opinion and feelings about it will also tend to cast things in a different light.

- **Manage your expectations of change and its impact**
  Because change is unsettling, it is tempting to make assumptions and presumptions about what will happen and the impact of the proposed changes. Wherever possible, try to ground your opinions in facts and figures and manage your expectations of what the likely outcome and longer-term impact will be.

- **Healthy body, healthy mind**
  You are more likely to have a positive outlook on change if you're looking after your body by eating a balanced diet, having regular exercise, getting quality rest and finding a healthy work-life balance. This provides a strong foundation on which to prepare for the uncertainty of change.

LEAVING HOME FOR THE FIRST TIME

There are lots of reasons why you might be leaving home for the first time: perhaps you're off to university or perhaps you have decided to move in with a partner or friend. Of course, not all of the reasons for leaving home might be positive; you might want to reduce conflict with your parents or other family members or want to move to a new area to feel more settled and safe.

Regardless of why you're leaving home, you're bound to be feeling a little nervous or overwhelmed and certainly a little excited too, which can have an effect on your mental health.

There is a lot you can do to stay in control and maintain your emotional wellbeing at this time of change:

- **Don't rush things:** As tempting as it might be to get to your new place as quickly as possible, take a moment to ensure that you can afford the move. The negative impact on your mental health could be significant if you boomerang back to where you started. And if you were motivated to move out because of family tensions, think about whether the issues can be resolved ahead of your move so that you don't leave on bad terms, if you can help it.

- **Ask for (and listen to) a few opinions:** Talk through your plans with friends or family members. They might have been in a similar situation themselves and could offer some valuable advice on how to make this work. They might offer a totally fresh and independent outlook.

- **Planning, planning, planning:** Think about the practicalities of moving to a new place. What will you need in terms of furnishings and furniture? What will be the cost of living and how will you subsidise this? Have you got a budget and are you confident when it comes to budgeting? Although you'll likely feel excited and emotional, it's important to be as practical and realistic as possible to ensure you minimize any future problems or challenges.

- **Give yourself a break:** Although you can be organized, it's realistic that you might feel homesick or lonely, especially in the first few days and weeks. How could these feelings be minimized? Will you be getting a job in the local area, are there any organizations or clubs you could join to meet new people? Who else do you know locally?

- **Keep in touch:** Hearing a friendly and familiar voice will help to reduce any feelings of homesickness, so try and set up regular calls with people at home. But don't be too reliant on home visits and keeping in touch, as it could reduce the time you've got to meet new people in your new community.

- **Make your house your home:** You'll feel more settled if you make sure that you've unpacked all your boxes and made this new space your own.

- **Put yourself out there:** Don't expect to meet new people or make new friends if you're sat indoors on your own. To extend your social circle in your new community you will need to get out, so join some clubs, sign up for a new sport, find a hobby, go to the pub or get out there to explore the local area.

A positive frame of mind is essential to help make leaving home for the first time a great experience. It's a huge milestone in anyone's life, but hopefully by following some of the steps here, you can help to ensure it's a change that works for you.

"Leaving home for the first time was the beginning of the new me. Prior to this I suffered depression and feelings of no self-worth. I think a new challenge is always good just to keep things fresh and exciting."

MENTAL HEALTH AND FURTHER EDUCATION

University or college is a fabulous opportunity to experience new things and make new friends and for many of us, further education is the first time that we move out of home and stand on our own two feet. But, of course, all this change in one go can be very overwhelming and for some of us, it can have a massive impact on our mental health.

In fact, a recent survey highlighted that more than one quarter (27%) of UK students reported having a mental health problem of one type or another. Here, female students were more likely than male students to have mental health problems (34% versus 19%) and LGBT students were at even higher risk than their heterosexual counterparts (45% versus 22%).[39]

Sadly, suicide is also becoming more prevalent at university with data revealing that the suicide rates among UK students had risen by 56% in the ten years between 2007 and 2017.[40]

To begin the process of reversing this trend, it's essential to consider mental health when embarking on further education. There are positive actions that can help:

- **Stay connected to your previous life:** Although you have lots of new adventures and experiences ahead, it's important to stay in touch with friends and family from home. As well as really understanding you, this important network is always there, particularly during difficult times, so don't forget they're there if you need them.

- **Don't hide away in your room:** You might feel daunted when it comes to meeting new people, but don't be tempted to hide in your room. It can be scary meeting new people, but prop your door open and say 'hello' to anyone wandering past or head down to the common room and be sociable. You're not on your own, in fact you're all in the same boat, so it might be reassuring to think that they're probably feeling as daunted as you are!

- **It's normal to feel homesick:** Homesickness can't be helped and when faced with a new home, new neighbours, a new environment and new challenges, it's normal to feel this way at some point. Keeping in touch with family and friends from home, as well as remembering that your fellow students are probably feeling the same way, is a good source of comfort that can help to overcome these feelings.

- **Keep yourself active:** A key part of looking after your mental health is looking after your physical health, so don't forget to keep active. As well as improving your mood and how you feel about yourself, exercise is also a great way to meet new people, so sign up for some sports clubs and societies.

- **Don't be too hard on yourself:** Further education is supposed to be challenging, so don't panic if you find it is stretching you. Manage your expectations of yourself; you're only just starting out, so don't expect to know everything in the first week! You'll be gradually working towards the qualification you're aiming for. The most important thing is to know who to ask for help, whether that's your tutor, a student counsellor or a fellow student.

- **Look for support when you need it:** If you are struggling with college or university, look around for the support that is there for you. Most further education providers will have counsellors or student support services, as well as learning support services that can help with any course questions or problems that you may have. The student union will also be able to advise and provide support, should you need it.

- **Be prepared to be assertive:** Living with new people in halls or a student house is a unique experience that can require a lot of patience and understanding from everyone involved. You need to be prepared to be assertive if the situation demands it and stand your ground on things like respecting each other's living space, as well as sharing the washing up and keeping communal areas relatively tidy and hygienic!

- **Plan your time to minimize stress:** To help ensure that you're not feeling under pressure with the study, sport and social life that you've got on your plate, it's important to plan your time. Try to make time to relax and recharge so that when things do get busy, for example when exam season starts, you're not feeling too under pressure.

- **Grab every opportunity you're presented with:** There is more to further education than being in a classroom or tutor group, so get out and take every opportunity available. As well as the opportunity to try something new, experiences and adventures that clubs, societies and work experience give will enhance your CV and give you a fresh outlook on life.

"Looking back on going to university, I don't think I was equipped to cope with all the change that becoming a student away from home brought. I remember feeling overwhelmed, getting to know housemates, a new routine, lots of new demands and expectations. Planning my time helped me to feel more in control. I learned that my housemates were all in the same position too, and they're a great support network one shouldn't overlook."

MENTAL HEALTH AND GRADUATION

Graduating from university or college is a significant milestone in life; it's the start of new things to come and a new life but also a moment to say goodbye to the lifestyle and community that you have become so comfortable with.

Managing this substantial change is certainly a challenge and it's easy to feel under pressure to deal with all the different decisions and changing circumstances that we just can't avoid any longer.

Some things you might have to deal with at this time include:

- **Dealing with your degree:** Have you been awarded the degree that you expected? There may be feelings of disappointment if you didn't achieve the qualification or level that you were anticipating. Or you may have unexpected decisions to take if you have achieved a higher grade than expected.

- **Managing your finances:** It's an unfortunate reality that many people graduate from higher education with significant student debts. Whilst many student loans won't need to be repaid until you've reached a certain income level, it's important to be aware of and in control of your personal finances.

- **Moving back home or to a new area:** If you haven't yet decided on your career post-graduation, you might find yourself living back at home with your parents which can mean stress and anxiety levels rocket. Alternatively, you might be moving to a new area which can present challenges of its own. Remembering some of the things you did when you started further education, in terms of making connections and getting out and about, will put you in good stead.

- **Starting a new job:** A new job is an exciting yet potentially overwhelming adventure, especially if it's your first 'real' job after graduation. You're bound to be nervous, but harness this energy into making it the best possible experience it can be: manage your expectations, ask lots of questions and bear in mind lots of the advice we share to protect your mental health mentioned throughout this book.

- **Planning your future:** You might have a clear plan about what you'd like to do going forward. You might want to travel the world, start a career or just take a break. But there's a good chance that you won't have a clue what you want to do with your life. This is OK and don't worry, it's completely normal! Take a moment, take a breath and let yourself dream big. You have a fantastic opportunity to live your best life, so don't rush into anything you're not sure about!

All of these considerations and decisions are potential causes of stress. But fortunately, there are a few simple steps to ensure you're in the best possible mental shape to cope.

- **Keep in touch:** Staying in touch with classmates will help you feel grounded and reassured that you're not alone. This will help transition you into a new life whilst ensuring that you retain support of the friends and connections that you've already nurtured.

- **Build and maintain a routine:** Introducing organization and routine into your post-education life is important to feeling good about yourself. Make sure to incorporate time to think about your goals and plans, as well as finding time to eat well and stay active. Your mental health definitely won't be helped if you're sat on the sofa, binge-watching TV and eating rubbish with the curtains closed!

- **Seek out the support that is available:** Depending on what you might be struggling with, there is support, advice and information out there. You might need more structured career advice or need to talk with a counsellor or healthcare professional about your mental health and how you're feeling. Whatever it is, make sure you talk about it and get your feelings back under control.

MENTAL HEALTH AND A NEW JOB

No matter how old or what stage of life you're at, when you start a new job it can feel overwhelming and daunting. This can contribute to stress and perhaps feelings of anxiety. In the days leading up to starting, your mind may be occupied with the challenges your new job will present and what your new colleagues and workplace will be like. At night your wandering mind might mean you have trouble sleeping.

Of course, a certain degree of stress is a good thing and it can help to keep you on your toes. When it comes to a new job that you're excited about, your adrenaline will be pumping, your heart will race a bit and it will help you to feel happy and energized.

Recognizing that these feelings are, for the most part, due to your changing circumstances and taking some positive steps to stay in control will help to ensure that your mental health isn't impacted by this new step on your career path.

- **Organize your life as much as possible:** This will ensure that your mornings aren't chaotic and being organized will help you to feel in control. Getting clothes ready for work the next day, making lunch and ensuring you have everything you need for the new challenges ahead is important.

- **Don't neglect your physical health:** Keep an eye on your food intake and make sure you eat a balanced diet. Alongside this, make sure you're not ignoring the importance of exercise and staying active. These have a huge impact on your performance in the workplace and will be a great way to manage your mental health.

- **Do what you can to get plenty of sleep and rest:** It's natural to struggle with falling asleep in the nights leading up to a new job. Follow some of the advice in the 'Getting a good night's sleep' chapter and remember how important rest and recovery is to keep you at your best.

- **Don't be afraid to ask for help:** It might be useful to ask for help from those around you to make the adjustment to your new routine as straightforward as possible. Be open with people about the help required and put some strategies in place to cope with, for example, any childcare emergencies that might arise.

As well as doing what you need to do to ensure you're in the best place to start a new job, you also need to be clear with your new employer about their expectations of you in your new role.

If you have questions about the company and your team, note them down so you don't forget them and raise them during your induction. And if something isn't clear, don't be afraid to ask. You spend a lot of your waking time in the office so it's vital that you're settled and feel comfortable in your new environment and role, as well as with your new team.

It's worth thinking about the reasons why you have made the decision to start a new job. If the reasons for the change were stress, workload pressures and a demanding boss, you need to be in the right frame of mind to ensure that this doesn't happen again.

Because of this, starting a new job is a fantastic opportunity to re-set your work/life balance. You might have found yourself at the mercy of a long hours culture at your last workplace, bringing work home with you regularly or finding yourself checking emails around the clock. A new job is a chance to make a fresh start which will pay you dividends when it comes to your mental health in the future.

MENTAL HEALTH AND PARENTHOOD

!!!

There are lots of online and offline resources and experts who can help when it comes to the demands of parenthood and the numerous questions that you are likely to have when you're caring for a little one, as well as yourself and your family. This chapter talks about the importance of nurturing positive mental health when you become a parent and should be considered alongside the very many other sources of support that are available to you.

There is a lot to think about when becoming a parent and often mental health isn't a priority, despite the fact that parenthood puts a lot of pressure on individuals and families. And although there are nine months to prepare for becoming a parent, there's no doubt that welcoming a new baby into the family can be a shock to the system relating to a range of feelings, including:

- Feeling trapped when you realize that there's no way back and life really has changed forever

- Dealing with the sleepless nights which can seem endless but, please believe, they do pass

- Coping with the constant demands of a baby or toddler, whether it's for food, nappies, sleep or attention, there's probably always something

- Guilt that you're not successfully balancing parenthood with all the other demands on your time, whether that's your relationship, family life, social life, work pressures or responsibilities in the home

- Unhappiness with your physical health, especially if you're the one who's carried the baby during pregnancy, as well as finding time to incorporate exercise and physical activity into your schedule

Coping with these feelings and emotions can inevitably have a negative impact on mental health, but a key approach to ensuring that things don't become too much is to re-frame experiences and invest time to adopting and nurturing a positive mindset.

- **Keep yourself active:** Physical health and fitness are important for life, but they are also a significant element of parenthood and promoting positive mental health. Take one day at a time and think about where physical activity can be incorporated into the new lifestyle.

- **Organization and routine will help you to feel in control:** And whilst you can't influence everything and there will be days when things don't go to plan, a routine will create a beneficial sense of comfort and security for you, your family and those around you. It also helps you to realize that you can't always do everything and that sometimes you need to say 'no' and schedule time to rest.

- **Keep talking and sharing:** At the early stages of parenting, it's easy to let talking and communicating with your partner slide. You're too tired, which makes you irritable and there's often a feeling that one of you (let's be honest, that's you!) is taking on the lion's share of the work. But you're in this together and you're a team, so share your feelings and remember to listen to each other.

- **Give yourself a break:** It's easy to assume that everyone else in the world has got parenting sussed. You only need to scroll through social media to be presented with countless images of perfect 'happy families' which, let's face it, isn't great for morale or motivation. Manage your social media use and take on board some of the advice in the two chapters relating to social media because the impressions given are not always the reality and shouldn't be something that you measure yourself and your worth against.

- **Remember that you're still you:** Having a child, whether you're a mum or a dad, doesn't take away anything from the person you were before, it just adds a new dimension to your story and personality. It might take a little while to come to terms with the change, but keep in mind that you are still you, you've just taken on a new role and challenge that will keep you on your toes for years to come!

"My husband had a particularly bad period with his mental health when our son was smaller and going through the tantrums stage was extremely hard for both of us. I needed his support, which he was unable to give me. There were times where I had to be both parents and deal with two situations simultaneously – the tantrum from my son and the anxiety from my husband. This was very hard, but I coped. Seeing someone you love suffer with mental health issues helped me to centre myself and deal with the situations."

MENTAL HEALTH AND AN EMPTY NEST

When a young person moves out of the family home, it's sometimes the case that the adults left behind experience what's known as 'empty nest syndrome'. Whilst this doesn't affect everyone, when it does hit it can bring with it feelings of sadness, grief and loneliness, and when these persist, they can, in extreme cases, develop into depression.

For women, whose lives have been particularly focused on childcare and managing the home, empty nest syndrome can be particularly hard to manage. But men aren't excluded from this and one study found that men also felt emotionally unprepared when a child left home, regretting the missed opportunities to be involved in their child's life.[41]

Here are a number of strategies to help cope with some of the challenges that an empty nest presents:

- **Minimize worry about those who have flown the nest:** You can alleviate some of the worry about your child leaving home by ensuring that they're ready for their new life. Whether it's being reassured that they can put a load of laundry on, that they know where the supermarket is and how to cook a simple meal and, importantly, that they know how to wash up!

- **Plan to keep in touch:** When your child has moved out, it's a chance to build a different and new relationship with them. You can still be close by staying in touch regularly by phone or messaging, so don't panic that you're not going to see or hear from them!

- **Recognize the opportunity:** Your new set-up at home gives you the opportunity to spend more time with your partner or friend or to take up a new activity or hobby. Consider some of the positive consequences of this change but, if you can only think about the down side, take a moment to consider how to re-frame the negatives into positives.

If you are struggling with an empty nest, you can also think about who you know that has been in a similar situation. Can you talk with a friend or neighbour whose children have also recently left home? Talking through your experiences could support you both to get through this time and they might suggest some ways that will help you deal with how you're feeling. And if you feel that you need more professional support, don't hesitate to talk with your doctor or approach a counsellor to discuss how you're feeling.

MENTAL HEALTH AND THE MENOPAUSE

The menopause is a natural part of the ageing process and usually occurs when we're between 45 and 55 years old as our oestrogen levels decline. Most women experience menopausal symptoms which can include hot flushes, night sweats, difficulty sleeping, poor moods, anxiety, reduced libido, vaginal dryness and problems with memory and concentration.[42]

The physical and emotional changes that the menopause brings can cause stress and anxiety among women and, in some cases, contribute to depression. This, combined with other life-changing events at this time of life, such as dealing with an empty nest, means that some women can feel isolated, lonely and struggling to cope.

Fortunately, there is much you can do to help yourself at this time. Making an appointment with your doctor is a great place to start as they may want to rule out any other physical conditions, such as thyroid problems, before confirming that you are going through menopause.

Your doctor may prescribe hormone replacement therapy or antidepressant medications to help you manage your menopause symptoms. But once you have sought some medical advice, there are some positive things you can do to support your mental health as you go through this change.

- **Review your sleep habits:** If the menopause is causing you restless nights, review your sleeping habits and see if there is anything you can do to improve the quality and amount of sleep that you're getting. Small changes, such as going to bed at the same time each night and setting an alarm for the same time each morning might help, as well as ensuring that your bedroom is dark, cool and quiet. You can see some more sleep advice in the 'Getting a good night's sleep' chapter.

- **Exercise is good for you:** As well as relieving the symptoms of stress, regular activity and exercise will aid sleep, boost mood and self-esteem. Advice for moving and getting active can be found in the 'Movement, exercise and mental health' chapter. A combination of cardio exercise such as walking, swimming, or tennis, as well as muscle-strengthening activity, such as yoga or weight-based workouts, are great for good physical health during the menopause.

- **Relax and recharge regularly:** Combat the feelings of stress during the menopause with activities such as yoga, meditation or tai chi, balanced with getting a bit of 'me' time like a massage or other types of pampering. Investing in yourself can also help if you're struggling with sleep and need more rest.

- **Find support from others in the same boat:** It's likely that some of your friends or family members will have been through or are going through menopause and they will be a great source of support and reassurance. Additionally, there may be local support groups where you can share your experiences with other women and make new friends in the process!

MENTAL HEALTH AND RELATIONSHIP BREAKDOWN

Just as we change and develop over time, so do our relationships and we shouldn't expect things to always be the way they were. When a relationship breaks down, it's inevitable that it will have an effect on our mental health and how we're feeling.

We might be feeling a loss, betrayal, anger, sadness, disappointment, grief, guilt or even relief. Each relationship is unique and as such the response to any break-up will be unique. That said, there is much you can do to protect and promote your mental health at this challenging time.

- **Give yourself time to adjust to the change:** Transitioning to a new life and a new way of living will be challenging and it will take time. It's unlikely that you will wake up the morning after a relationship breakdown and move on immediately so it's important not to pretend that you will. At the same time by continuing to dwell on what's happened and not looking forward to the future, you'll find it difficult to adjust to the change. So make sure to focus on the good things that are bound to come.

- **Don't look back:** It might be tempting to rely on your ex-partner for support, if that's something you're used to doing, but it's important to try and resist. You need to focus on the future and building your own strength and resilience; things have changed, and you need to maintain the space that your break-up has naturally created.

- **Focus on the positives:** Although you may be feeling down, try and visualize the future as you'd like to see it. Keep this vision in mind, perhaps write it down or make a sketch to remind yourself and refer back to it if you find yourself struggling.

- **Make sure you look after you:** Your resilience and mental health will certainly be improved if you focus on your physical wellbeing, which includes your diet, hydration, sleep and exercise. Be mindful that you're not relying on things like alcohol, drugs or food to cope with your feelings and, if you think you are, be strong enough to admit that you might need some help from an expert.

- **Get out and find something to do:** While you're coming to terms with things, getting out and about and enjoying a favourite sport or activity is a great way to keep your mood positive. You might want to have a walk and a chat with a friend or arrange to go for lunch or coffee with someone you've not seen for ages.

- **Find someone to talk to and let your feelings out:** It's important to talk with someone about what has happened and how you're feeling. This might be a friend or family member or, if it's easier, a healthcare professional or counsellor. You'll be experiencing a range of emotions and you'll benefit from talking through them and, in time, creating a positive plan for the future.

Be reassured that you will move on in time – it's a cliché but time is a great healer! – and that you don't have to deal with any of this on your own. But if you find that your emotions aren't changing and you're not feeling more positive, it could be the sign of an underlying mental health issue and, if this is the case, you really need to speak up and ask for some professional help and support.

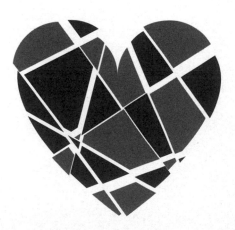

PART 5

YOUR MENTAL HEALTH AT WORK

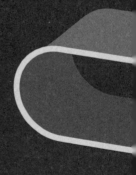

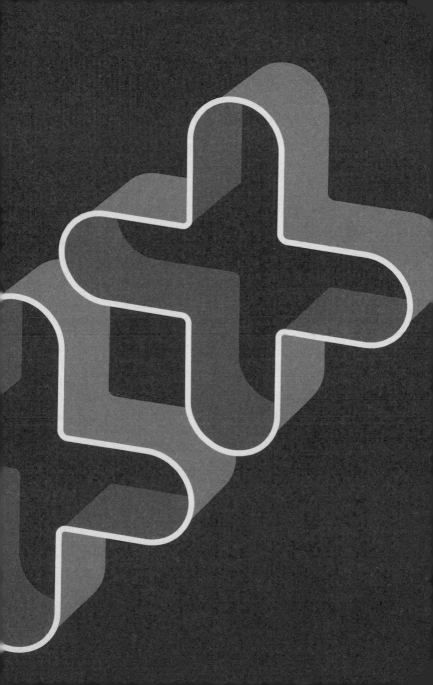

FEEL REASSURED THAT YOUR MENTAL HEALTH IS PROTECTED BY LAW

Even though your employer might be totally on board with promoting positive mental health in the workplace, it's reassuring to know that mental health is also protected by law.

Of course, the protection that the law offers to employees with mental health issues does depend on the geographic location of your employer, but there are, for example, legal requirements in the UK for employers to ensure that employees have a safe place to work, with support if issues occur.

Most of these laws require that organizations protect an individual's psychological and physical health 'as far as reasonably practicable'. Health and Safety legislation highlights the importance of identifying and minimizing risks, and all organizations need to have a clear policy on this, including provisions for psychosocial risks.

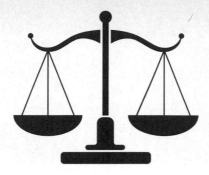

More widely, mental health is all about valuing differences, and many national laws state that employers should not discriminate based on 'protected' characteristics such as age, disability, gender reassignment, marriage or civil partnership, pregnancy and maternity, race, religion or belief, gender and sexual orientation.

If you are treated unfairly due to you having a protected characteristic or you are helping a friend or family friend who has one, this is likely to be unlawful and you should seek clarification of how your national law is structured to help your respond.

WORK IS GOOD FOR YOUR MENTAL HEALTH!

Work can have a positive impact on our health and general wellbeing. Organizations simply operate better when we, the employees, are physically and mentally healthy.

Mental health is integral to how you feel about your job, how you perform and how you interact with management, colleagues and customers. Employers need to know that employees who have good mental health are more likely to perform well, have good attendance and be fully engaged in their work.

It's an argument that's been backed up by government research confirming that work provides the resources for material wellbeing, but also meets important psychosocial needs, enhancing individuals' identity and social status.[43]

A few things you can do to ensure that work positively influences your mental health include:

- **Learn to say no:** Make sure you understand your capabilities, and recognize that the better you manage your time, the better your chances of avoiding an excessive work overload. Only you will know when *possible* turns into *impossible* – one key skill to manage workplace stress and the huge variety of demands is to say 'no' when you should, and at the earliest opportunity. You may be tempted to take on more work than you can handle to win praise or recognition, but in the long term you might be asking for trouble.

- **Build a positive relationship with your boss:** A positive, two-way relationship with your supervisor can be crucial in helping to manage your workload, and facilitating a conversation about resolving the issues that may affect your mental health. Even if there isn't an issue now, the foundations of a strong relationship will ensure you can start a conversation as and when the need arises.

- **Establish some boundaries:** In the modern-day workplace we're reachable almost anytime, anywhere, which means it's vital to set boundaries. Try to leave work on time and try to resist checking or responding to work emails after hours. Certainly don't check them before bed, over the weekend or while you're on leave.

You'll have a strong sense of what you need to do and it's not likely that you'll want or need to do everything at the same time. Do what you think feels achievable and applicable, but small, positive steps will make a lasting difference.

CREATING A WORK ENVIRONMENT THAT SUPPORTS MENTAL HEALTH

There are some positive steps you can take to help ensure that your work environment is one that sustains and supports both mental and physical health:

- **Be aware of negative or judgemental terminology and language:** Challenge this whenever you witness it, making sure to address gossip or negative behaviours immediately and directly. This will help create a workplace culture that does not tolerate harassment or discrimination.

- **Regularly and consistently encourage and promote healthy work-life practices:** Are there ways you can help promote an environment where everyone takes advantage of flexible hours, job sharing or working from home? Can you encourage healthy eating or physical activity among your co-workers? Are you going home at a reasonable time, taking the holidays that you've earned and taking any other time off that is owed to you? You shouldn't be expected to check work emails at home, so make it a habit not to do this.

- **Think about whether your workplace recognizes, appreciates and rewards achievement:** Do you and your colleagues feel good about what you do for a living? Are you confident in your ability to offer honest and objective feedback at work, taking the opportunity to learn from your mistakes when they do happen?

- **Encourage and support a work environment that promotes openness, understanding and respect for mental health issues:** Can you talk with your colleagues in a matter-of-fact way about mental health? And if they are struggling with this, do you treat them the same as you would if you were talking about any other workplace concern?

WHAT CAN YOUR EMPLOYER BE DOING TO HELP?

Because work is so intrinsically linked to our mental health, it is important for an employer to take positive steps to improve mental health in the workplace, to tackle the causes of work-related mental ill health, create a workplace culture where employees feel able to talk about their mental health and support those who are experiencing mental ill health.

A forward-thinking employer will have a clearly defined policy to help ensure that they take a consistent and considered approach to mental health in the workplace, as well as highlighting the organization's dedication and commitment to promoting positive mental health.

In reality this will include:

- A published statement of the organization's commitment to promoting positive mental health for all employees and tackling the causes of work-related mental ill health. This should come from the top of an organization – the higher the better – and should communicate the company's vision for creating a workplace where all employees feel able to talk openly about their mental health without fear of stigma or discrimination

- A requirement for all managers and employees to receive mental health training

- Recognition that an employee's performance or behaviour might be affected if they experience mental health issues. This reassures employees that, if mental health issues appear, appropriate support and accommodations will be explored

- A request for employees to seek help at the earliest opportunity, with the knowledge that their employer will do their best to support them

- A process to reintegrate employees who have been absent from work due to mental health issues back into the workplace

- Signposting for employees and managers, directing them to more information and support on questions, issues and organizations relating to mental health and wellbeing

You might also find it useful to reflect on how and what your employer is doing when it comes to supporting and nurturing your mental health.

- How do you think they are doing when it comes to identifying and tackling the causes of mental ill health in your workplace?

- What activities are they organizing to educate staff and management about mental health?

- Has training been offered to raise awareness of the signs and symptoms of mental ill health?

If you feel your employer needs to improve their support systems, you should take the opportunity to highlight what you think needs to be put in place. After all, the organization has a legal 'duty of care' towards you and your mental health.

"I have had referrals to occupational health and counselling through work. Now, looking back, I needed to embrace the offer but because I was in poor mental health I didn't really open up to the experience."

Making an appointment with your doctor is a great place to start.

CAN A WELLNESS RECOVERY ACTION PLAN HELP YOU?

Wellness Recovery Action Plans (WRAPs) were created by Mary Ellen Copeland, an author, educator and mental health recovery advocate in the US. Many organizations have adopted a WRAP to help managers and employees proactively support mental health and wellbeing in the workplace.

This tool is a way for an employer to show you their commitment to wellbeing, whether it's for the benefit of a new or current employee in the process of working through a mental health issue.

WRAPs cover a range of things, including:

- Methods that an individual can use to support their own mental wellbeing
- Warning signs for emerging mental health issues
- Workplace triggers for poor mental health
- Line manager and workplace support strategies for mental health

A WRAP is an informal, confidential agreement between an employee and the employer to promote wellbeing. It's a document that will evolve and develop as things change for the employee, and they should take the responsibility to write and own it, expressing personal preferences, choices and needs relating to mental health and general wellbeing. It is also best written in positive mental health so early signs of mental health deterioration can be highlighted to enable prompt action to be taken.

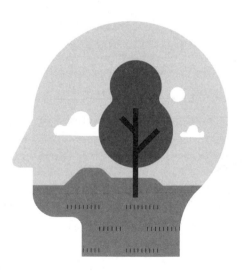

QUESTIONS TO CONSIDER
WHEN PREPARING A WRAP

What things, situations or people help you
to stay mentally healthy at work?

What support can your manager offer to help
you stay mentally healthy at work?

Are there any specific situations at work
that trigger poor mental health?

How would poor mental health impact
your performance at work?

Are there any early warning signs that
your manager or colleagues could spot
that your mental health is suffering?

What support could your manager put
in place to help you manage these triggers
and symptoms of poor mental health?

What should your manager or colleagues do
if you do experience mental health issues?

OPENING UP ABOUT YOUR MENTAL HEALTH IN THE WORKPLACE

It's a big deal to open up and talk about mental health issues with anyone when you're feeling anxious or distressed, but particularly with colleagues and managers. Often, it is tempting to believe it's easier to continue with the struggle, rather than reaching out for help and letting someone in on what's going on.

In reality, there is no going back after opening up to another person about mental health issues and this is something that many people don't feel able to do. In Britain, 38% of workers admit they wouldn't talk openly about a mental health problem for fear that it would affect their job prospects or job security.[44]

But it is worth considering that – as obvious as it sounds – the sooner mental health concerns are tackled, the sooner positive change will be made.

Before talking with your manager or a colleague, take a moment to put yourself in their shoes: they are likely to be as nervous as you are about having this type of conversation.

As a result, they might come across reluctant to talk or might appear 'cold' because they're nervous about saying the wrong thing or responding in the 'wrong' way.

This isn't your problem, it's theirs. Although it's necessary to bear it in mind, their discomfort isn't something you have any control over and therefore shouldn't be something you worry about.

However, the more open and honest you can be, the better the long-term outcome will be for you, the employer and the wider team. By sharing the background of the problem, you will help them to offer better support, advice and information in return.

It's important to know that you should not be treated badly at work because of a mental health condition. Under the Equality Act (2010), employers in the UK have a legal duty to make 'reasonable adjustments' and not discriminate in recruiting, retaining or promoting staff. Mental health conditions and problems are a disability under this legislation and employers should work in partnership with an employee to deliver on this duty.

When opening up to your manager, there are some practical elements associated with talking to them about your mental health that should be considered:

- **How do you want to broach the subject of a meeting?:** Are you more comfortable emailing or asking face-to-face for a meeting? Email is fine but be aware of adding too much personal information in an email or using it as a way to 'let off steam'. It is impossible to take it back once you press send, and the contents of a note can easily be misunderstood and misinterpreted.

- **Be clear what you are asking for:** Request a one-to-one meeting with your manager. Explain that you would like the opportunity to discuss some issues you've been grappling with and how they relate to your work. Discuss the support your manager can offer to help you manage your mental health and enable you to perform better.

- **Is there a location for the meeting that you would prefer?:** Where will you be most comfortable discussing these matters? And would you prefer to meet with your manager alone, or would you like a trade union representative or a colleague to be present too?

Ahead of talking at such a meeting, take the time to consider how much you want to share and how the challenges you're experiencing can be best framed. Here are some considerations to put your mental health issues into context and prepare for reactions you may receive.

- Is the cause of your mental health condition related to your personal or home life? What background and information on this are you prepared to share?

- Has there been a specific incident or situation at work that has exacerbated the problem? Or have things been building up over time?

- How much information do you want to share? Do you want to request complete confidentiality? If talking with your line manager, decide together, which colleagues, if any, should be informed and what they would be told

- Opening up and acknowledging mental health issues is an emotional experience. How will you manage these feelings during the meeting?

- Is there something that managers or colleagues could do to reduce stress or minimize the impact of your mental health condition?

- What support is there from the organization to help mental health? This might be via your employer-funded EAP or Occupational Health team

- What is the company's sick pay policy? Can you self-certify your absence, if it's required, for a period of time or will you need to produce a note from your doctor?

- Is there a benefit to putting your doctor directly in touch with your employer? Or would this make you more anxious?

- How is this meeting going to be followed up? Is there a way to track progress on the issues raised or monitor how you are feeling about things?

Once an employer is aware of your mental health issues, they have a legal obligation to support you. Meeting with them is the first step in seeking help. What happens next will be guided by your manager. Let them confirm what follow-up will take place, the timeline and what you can expect as the next steps.

But don't forget that the company's 'duty of care' does not replace your responsibility to look after yourself the best you can. This includes actively helping yourself in whatever ways possible.

SUPPORTING A COLLEAGUE'S MENTAL HEALTH

We spend a lot of time with work colleagues and as such we have an opportunity to play an important role if we suspect that they may be struggling with their mental health. But the sensitive nature of mental health means that it can be difficult for a colleague to open up, so we should be careful about how we approach it.

Sometimes, it might be immediately obvious when someone is struggling with mental health issues and you can take swift action to help them. Other times you might gradually spot the signs and symptoms, perhaps over a period of weeks or months.

When the time feels right to approach a co-worker about your concern for them and their mental health, it's important that the conversation is proactive, positive and supportive. Here are some tips to help ensure that it is:

- **Choose the right place to talk:** Where you decide to talk about mental health needs should be quiet and private, so the person feels comfortable and equal.

A location outside the workplace may work well, and if they work from home, you might want to meet with them there, on their territory.

- **Encourage people to talk with you:** People can find it difficult to talk about their mental health, but they are likely to feel less reluctant if workplace conversations about these matters are normalized, seen and heard on a regular basis.

- **Use simple, open and non-judgemental questions:** These will enable people to explain what they think the problem is, how it manifests itself, what the triggers are, how it affects their work and home life, and what support would help them overcome these challenges.

- **Don't be tempted to make assumptions:** It's easy to guess the symptoms a colleague might have and how these are affecting their ability to do their job. But don't assume anything! Let them tell you how they can best manage their mental health and the support they would like from you.

- **Listen to what you're told:** Everyone's experience with a mental health problem is different, so don't be tempted to think there's a 'one size fits all' solution. Have a flexible approach to offering help and advice, remembering that what might be right for you won't always be right for someone else.

- **Assure the employee of confidentiality:** People need to be reassured that what they have shared will be treated with confidence. Discuss precisely what information they want to be shared and be sure that any subsequent third-party conversations are in line with the latest data protection legislation.

- **Encourage them to get professional advice and support:** Encourage them to talk with their doctor about the struggles they're having, as well as other support services, such as EAP or Occupational Health services.

Continue to reassure the colleague that your concern is sincere and that you're ready, willing and able to talk with them. If the time for the conversation arrives and the person decides that the moment isn't right, assure them that you'll be ready to help whenever they need you.

TIME OFF WORK FOR MENTAL HEALTH ISSUES

If you're absent from work because of a mental health problem – or a physical illness, for that matter – it is recommended to stay in touch with your employer and colleagues. This will help to address practical issues, such as sharing information about your recuperation and expected return-to-work dates, as well as keeping you connected to your team. Your manager and employer will provide the opportunity to address any concerns or worries you might have as they arise.

Keeping in touch prevents feeling isolated from colleagues because of an absence. Maintaining a connection with them and not cutting yourself off will make the transition back to work more comfortable for everyone.

While absent from work, it's natural to feel nervous and have lots of questions about the future, your job and what happens next.

Some things for you to think about include:

- Do you want to hear from work? Are you OK with management and colleagues sending cards, emailing or calling you to find out how things are going?

- If you do want people to keep in touch or visit, are there questions or topics that you'd prefer to keep off-limits? What will you do if someone does visit or call and veers into areas you'd rather not discuss?

- Can you arrange a time to pop into work for a cup of tea, to stay connected with your team and catch up on what's been going on?

- Is there a colleague who can keep in touch with you directly, let you know what is happening and relay your progress back to others at work?

- What support can your employer provide while you're absent from work? Are there counselling support, occupational health advice or healthcare services that can aid and assist in your recovery?

- Is there an opportunity to have a staggered return to work that would perhaps let you start off working a few hours a day from home?

- Are you worried about the security of your job? Or is your absence causing any financial problems for you? What support and reassurance can your employer offer to allay these fears?

Make note of any concerns and questions you have while you're away and raise them with your manager at the earliest opportunity so that worries don't fester. Your employer and co-workers will want you back at work quickly, but not until you're ready, so by keeping channels of communication open, you can make sure to update everyone on your recovery.

WHEN IT'S TIME TO RETURN TO WORK

Returning to work after taking time off for a mental health issue is a big step to take, just as it would be after taking time off to recuperate and recover from a physical condition.

When getting ready to return to work, a good starting point is to consider the support or adjustments that would help make the return a successful, long-term one.

There are a few questions to reflect on ahead of returning to work, including:

- Is there a particular aspect of the job that makes you feel stressed or anxious?

- Can you think of anything that could be done to address this and make a positive change?

- Depending on the timing of your return, is there a project, event or deadline that you might need more support to deliver on?

- Would it be useful to lighten your workload and delegate some duties and responsibilities to a colleague?

- Is there an opportunity to work from home or adjust your working hours so, for example, you're not travelling in to work during rush hour?

- Do you need any additional time off for more treatment or rehabilitation?

- What do you want colleagues to be told about the time you've been away?

- Are you ready for potentially uncomfortable or tactless questions about the time you've been away? How will you handle these?

- Is there extra training that might boost your skills or confidence?

- How do you want your progress to be monitored when you're back at work? How often do you want to meet with your manager to catch up, and where would you be most comfortable having these meetings?

- What steps can you take to minimize the possibility of your mental health deteriorating and the need to take time off in the future?

- Is there an opportunity to informally meet with a colleague ahead of your return, to break the ice and get back into the swing of things?

In preparing to return to work it is important to manage expectations of yourself, as it can take a while to settle back into to a 'normal' routine and you may initially feel more tired than normal. Do what you can to get ready for your return and remember that there are lots of people and support channels available if you need them.

WORKPLACE ADJUSTMENTS TO ENHANCE YOUR MENTAL HEALTH

Making adjustments in the workplace is important to help with mental health issues. These modifications can help reduce the length of time you're absent from work and help keep you there – feeling good and performing well – once you return.

The right adjustments will enable you to feel trusted, capable and empowered to do your job, and reassured that you're being supported by your employer.

Remember, you are the expert in how you're feeling, and you'll know best what changes, considerations and support you need. Communication is key to making the right changes, so with your manager discuss what you can and can't do and work in partnership to find appropriate solutions.

Whilst it might be tempting for an employer to micro-manage you when you're struggling with mental health issues and reduce your workload, this isn't the right thing to do. In fact, adopting this approach could actually be counterproductive – if work is not sufficiently challenging, people can lose motivation and feel disengaged from their work and employer.

Your sense of anxiety and mental distress might actually intensify if you feel your employer does not trust your ability to do the job.

Workplace adjustments that can practically support you don't have to be extravagant or complicated. Often the most effective changes are small and simple. Here are some that are worth discussing with your employer:

- Can flexible working hours or a change to your start or finish time make a difference? If you work shifts, can you change your shift pattern or your days off?

- What about changing your break or lunch times? Or you could ask for more frequent, shorter breaks throughout the working day

- Can adjustments be made to your physical workspace? Would somewhere quieter or a bit livelier help you adjust to work?

- Is there a quiet room in the workplace that you can access to get some privacy, or a 'safe space' where you can get some time out?

- Is there an opportunity for you to work from home? It's important that this doesn't have the effect of isolating you, so think about how you could do this whilst still staying connected with the organization and your colleagues

- Can your employer agree to give you time off for appointments relating to your mental health treatment, such as counselling sessions?

- Can some of your tasks be reallocated in the short term, or could changes be made to your duties? Alternatively, could you be redeployed to a different role?

- Is there additional training, support or mentoring that you could receive? This might include training to help you build your resilience and coping skills

- Can your manager offer you greater supervision or support? And can they offer you more feedback on your work, taking regular opportunities to discuss, review and reflect on your positive achievements?

Regardless of the adjustments that are put in place, it is important to revisit and reflect on the impact they're having. This will give you and your employer the opportunity to tweak and change them as required and ensure that the support put in place is effective.

CREATING A LONG-TERM PLAN FOR MANAGING MENTAL HEALTH IN THE WORKPLACE

Having an ongoing mental health condition doesn't mean that you aren't capable of continuing to work effectively and perform at a high level.

And, just as importantly, there is no reason why you should be treated differently because you have a mental health condition. It is not lawful for your employer to make assumptions about your capabilities based on your mental health issues and discriminate against you.

Most people with ongoing mental health issues continue to work successfully and not every case demands specific support from an employer. Where support is necessary, it is important that an employer is flexible and in agreement on what is required.

Established management performance review procedures, work planning and employees' individual needs should take into account your requirements if you have an on-going mental health issue. So, establish a positive relationship with your employer, one that leverages an open, two-way channel of communication. That can make all the difference, allowing you to discuss your progress and what they can do to help.

As part of your ongoing care and recovery, you will have been encouraged to develop coping strategies. These can be small things that can prevent longer-term absence or a deterioration in your mental health. One coping strategy might be to identify the signs of a possible relapse and take steps to avoid it. These might include prioritizing time to relax or adjust your work-life balance, as well as increasing the amount of exercise you get and cutting down on alcohol.

You could also talk with your employer about drafting an 'advance directive' or a WRAP. The chapter 'Can a Well-ness Recovery Action Plan help you?' outlines how you'd like to be treated in the workplace in the event that your mental health declines. Here you'd include information on the symptoms that management and colleagues should look out for, who can be contacted in the event of an issue and the type of support that would be helpful for you.

UTILIZING THE WEALTH OF EXPERTISE WITHIN YOUR ORGANIZATION

There are lots of different experts within each organization who can offer information and advice on mental health and wellbeing. Here is a run-down of the most common experts.

THE HUMAN RESOURCES TEAM

The Human Resources (HR) team within your organization has a pivotal role to play when it comes to identifying, supporting, protecting and nurturing mental health in the workplace.

Whether it is creating a mental health policy for the organization, designing and delivering training to employees and managers or ensuring compliance with legislation relating to mental health, wellbeing, disability and discrimination, HR is central to how mental health is discussed and 'normalised' within a workplace.

The HR team is also a strong internal resource to help managers support employees with mental health issues, either by ensuring that they're following established procedures and policies to support and manage employees or by acting as a sounding board for a manager's questions about these matters.

HR can direct an employee to the specialist support services that are in place to assist with mental health issues, as well as answer any questions you might have.

YOUR MANAGER

We've talked a lot about managers' involvement and it's important not to overlook or underestimate their role in supporting and protecting your mental health and wellbeing in the workplace.

Management provides an important channel for you to talk about mental health concerns and ask for advice on coping with stress and pressure in the workplace. Your manager will also monitor your work environment, performance and changes jointly agreed upon to support your mental health.

Managers are a conduit between you and the organization, looking out for signs of mental health issues and balancing the needs and priorities of all parties to ensure that you ultimately have the support, information and advice you need to stay keep mentally healthy in the workplace.

EMPLOYEE ASSISTANCE PROGRAMMES

An Employee Assistance Programme (EAP) is a workplace programme designed to assist with productivity and attendance issues, supporting employees by identifying and resolving personal concerns and issues that may be affecting job performance. These might include health, marital, family, financial, alcohol, drug, legal, emotional, stress or other personal issues.

An EAP acts as a gateway to a range of services and support, including:

- Counselling and other short-term psychological services
- Money advice and debt management
- Child- and elder-care information services
- Legal information and guidance
- Information on emotional, work-life and workplace issues
- Management referrals and support

An employee's use of an EAP service is voluntary and the vast majority of people who take advantage of them do so through self-referrals. As such, one of the most essential functions of an EAP is its ability to provide confidential support services, on demand, when they're needed and free of charge to employees.

EAPs accept referrals from other groups within an organization, including trade union representatives, HR professionals and managers. The specific way in which these referrals are managed depends on the company and will take into account the employer's HR policies, as well as data protection regulations.

The EAP delivers consultation and training for managers and supervisors within an organization, giving mangers the opportunity to discuss workplace issues and challenges they might be facing, and providing support and guidance on how to manage these situations in a constructive way.

Information on how to contact your organization's EAP will be available from your HR team or on your company's intranet.

OCCUPATIONAL HEALTH

Occupational Health services within an organization can support mental health and wellbeing in a number of ways, such as:

- Conducting health assessments to ensure that employees are fit to perform duties in the workplace, whether by statutory requirement or simply as a good employment practice. This is an important aspect of health, safety and wellbeing management

- Monitoring for signs of work-related ill health, enabling organizations to comply with current legislation and preventing mental and physical problems from developing This helps ensure that procedures are in place to effectively manage any health risks

- Offering management advice and support on employee performance and attendance matters, helping managers determine why an employee may have an issue with attendance and recommending the best support options, especially if mental health problems are a factor

- Providing management with information on health trends, underlying issues and areas for improvement when it comes to managing workplace health and wellbeing

Occupational Health professionals can also help with rehabilitation and provide advice, treatment and support that will help you to get back to work or get back to your expected performance levels as quickly as possible.

As well as those experts available within your organization, there are lots of national and international charities, organizations and experts who can offer support, advice and information on mental health. You can find out more about some of these experts in Part Six.

YOUR MENTAL HEALTH WHEN YOU'RE JOB-HUNTING

Discussing mental health with your manager can be a challenge when you're already working for an employer, but when looking for a new job, the question of whether to disclose these issues to a prospective employer can be a tough one to answer.

On the one hand, the more honest you are with a prospective employer, the better they can support you in managing your mental health. However, for many people it's not necessary to ask for or receive any specific support for their condition.

As a result, and due to the stigma still attached to mental health problems, sharing details of struggles is something that needs to be carefully considered.

Clearly, there isn't a right answer here and you might want to find out more about the organization and its employees before opening up about mental health issues you have or have had in the past.

The following questions might help you decide on the best course of action:

- How would disclosing your mental health issues impact your mental health? Would it take some pressure off, or would it create additional stress?

- Do you take any medication that has side effects that may influence your ability to do the job or work with others?

- Do you have enough information on what the job you're applying for entails?

- What do you know about the culture of the company or the team that you will be working with? Have you had an opportunity to meet them as part of the recruitment process?

- Do you think your mental health might impact your ability to do the job you're applying for?

- Would knowing about your mental health issues help management offer the support you need and make necessary accommodations?

You can also consider whether there is a positive aspect to your mental health issue that might benefit your job application. For example, can you provide examples of where your condition has given you better insight into supporting others or empathising with how they might be feeling? Or would it make you a better manager when it comes to supporting others who might be experiencing mental health issues?

If you do have mental health problems and decide not to tell your manager, you cannot expect them to work with you on managing your mental health.

Of course, if you do disclose a mental health condition to a prospective employer, employers in many countries cannot discriminate against current or potential employees on the basis of their disability. This legislation extends to the recruitment and retention, promotion and transfer, training and development, as well as dismissal of employees.

Here, 'disability' is defined as a physical or mental impairment that has a substantial and long-term adverse effect on a person's ability to carry out normal, day-to-day activities. Your mental health issue could be considered a mental impairment, and therefore your employer must also consider whether there is any type of support or accommodations they could make to enable you to do the job.

Lastly, the actual process of job hunting can be a stressful and demoralising time so why not look to put in place some of the advice included in this book to help you?

+PART 6
WHAT TO
DO NEXT?

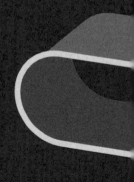

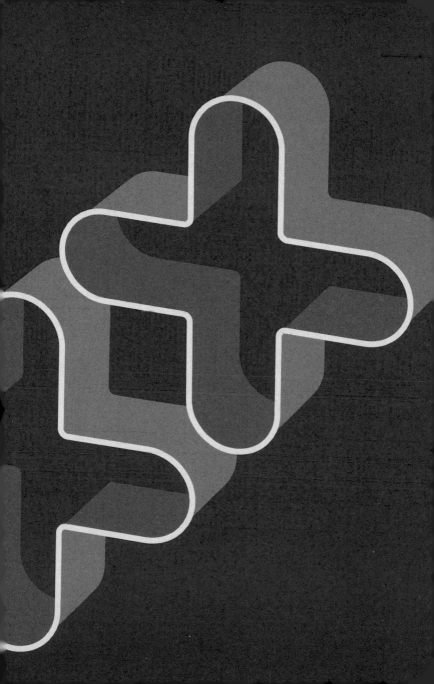

TEN TIPS TO ACHIEVE BETTER MENTAL HEALTH

Mental health is something we all 'have' and experience – it is very personal to us and changes throughout our lives as circumstances change. One in four adults and one in ten children experience a mental health issue during their life while many more of us know and care for people who do.

It is helpful to think of mental health on a scale and appreciate that we all have some days that are better than others. Where we are on one particular day does not define us.

An important part of keeping physically well and mentally healthy is to take care of yourself. There are plenty of things you can do. We've touched on each of these earlier, but here are our top ten tips to achieve better mental health.

1. Get plenty of sleep

Sleep is really important for good physical and mental health. Sleep helps regulate the chemicals in our brain that transmit information. These chemicals play a key role in managing our moods and emotions. If we don't get enough sleep, we can start to feel depressed or anxious.

Organizations such as The Sleep Foundation provide tips on how to overcome problems with sleeping.[45]

2. Eat well

Eating well is not just important for the body, but also for the mind.

Certain mineral deficiencies, such as iron and vitamin B12 deficiencies, can lead to poor moods. As such, aim to eat a balanced, healthy diet and drink plenty of water.

If you're a particularly stressed or anxious person, try limiting or cutting out caffeine, as it can make you feel jittery and anxious. And remember that caffeine is not just in coffee – tea, energy drinks, supplements, soft drinks and chocolate can all have caffeine in them, and often in higher quantities than you might think!

3. Avoid alcohol, smoking and drugs

Drinking alcohol and smoking can impact mental health.

Having too many drinks can result in feeling more depressed and anxious the next day as well as making it harder to concentrate. Excessive drinking for prolonged periods can also result in thiamine deficiency. Thiamine (vitamin B1) is important for good brain functioning and a deficiency can lead to severe memory problems, coordination problems, confusion and eye problems.

Withdrawal – the set of symptoms experienced when the use of medications or recreational drugs are decreased or discontinued – is known to be especially challenging for mental wellbeing. If you smoke, between cigarettes your body and brain go into withdrawal, which makes you irritable and anxious. Other drugs will leave you in withdrawal and can often cause very poor moods and anxiety.

More severe effects of drug use include paranoia and delusions. Some research suggests that drug use is related to the development of mental disorders like schizophrenia.

4. Get plenty of sunlight (but not too much!)

Sunlight is a great source of vitamin D, which is important for the body and the brain. It helps the brain release chemicals that improve our mood, like endorphins and serotonin.

Try to go out in the sun when possible, but make sure to keep your skin and eyes safe. Thirty minutes to two hours a day of sunlight is ideal. During the winter, some people become depressed because they aren't getting enough sunlight – this is known as Seasonal Affective Disorder (SAD). Some find that using a special light-therapy lamp helps to alleviate these symptoms.

5. Manage stress

Stress is often unavoidable but knowing what triggers stress and how to cope with it is key to maintaining good mental health. Try to manage your responsibilities and worries by making a list or a schedule of when you can resolve each issue.

Breaking down worries and stresses and noting them in a list will help you realize that often that they are manageable. Try to avoid burying your head in the sand and tackle problems face on. If you're having trouble sleeping or are waking up thinking about stressful things, it will help to write them down before going to sleep and reassuring yourself that these can be dealt with in the morning. So keep a pen and paper beside your bed to manage sleep time stress.

6. Do something you enjoy

Try to make time for doing the fun things you enjoy. If you like going for a walk with the dog, spending time with friends, painting or watching a certain TV show, try to set aside time for those activities and enjoy yourself. If we don't spend any time doing the things we enjoy, we can become irritable and unhappy.

7. Find time for physical activity and exercise

Activity and exercise are essential for maintaining good mental health.

Being active not only gives a sense of achievement, it also boosts the chemicals in the brain that help put you in a good mood. Exercising can help eliminate poor moods, anxiety, stress and feeling tired and disengaged.

You do not need to run a marathon or spend hours in the gym; a short walk or some other gentle activity often does the trick. Also, exercising with others, and sharing your worries and concerns along the way is often a good way of improving your mood.

8. Connect with others and be sociable
Make an effort to maintain good relationships and talk to people whenever you get the chance.

Having friends is important not just for your self-esteem, but also for providing support when you're not feeling too great. Research has found that talking to others for just ten minutes can actually improve memory and test scores.

9. Do things for others
Helping others is not just good for the people you're helping, it's good for you too.

Helping someone can boost self-esteem and make you feel good about your place in the world. Feeling as though you are part of a community is in fact a really important part of your mental health. Try volunteering for a local charity, or just being neighbourly.

10. Ask for help – and do not be embarrassed to do so

An important way to keep yourself mentally healthy is to recognize when you're not feeling good and know when to ask for help. There is no shame in asking someone for support if you're feeling low or stressed. Everyone goes through patches where they do not feel as good as they should.

Try speaking with friends or family, or if you think your mental health is in decline speak to your doctor or, if you have one, an EAP provider or occupational health adviser.

Individuals suffering from mental health problems have been stigmatized for centuries, and too many people – especially men

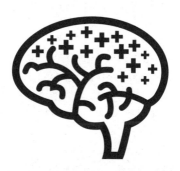

– have ended up not receiving any help at all. People of all ages have found themselves grappling with services that treat mind and body separately. This has led to hundreds of thousands of lives being put on hold or ruined and many thousands of tragic and unnecessary deaths.

But the future is looking brighter; in recent years the picture has started to change for the better. Public attitudes towards mental health have and are continuing to improve. There is a growing commitment among communities, workplaces, schools and across society to change the way we think about it.

To help change thinking on this important public health issue, please share these top tips – and ideally this book – with those who might need it.

You can and should be part of the movement to destigmatize mental health problems, raise awareness and give parity to mental health alongside physical health.

WHERE TO GO FOR HELP AND SUPPORT ON MENTAL HEALTH ISSUES

Your doctor is the first point of contact if you wish to access mental health services. In addition to assessing an individual's circumstances and offering appropriate treatment or advice, your doctor can refer you to a psychological therapy or specialist mental health service for further advice or treatment.

There may also be organizations that offer counselling, coaching or stress management courses. Getting to know what is available, and then plucking up the courage to make contact, is probably the hardest – but also the most important – step in moving forward.

A full guide to the mental health services available through the NHS is available online at **https://www.nhs.uk/NHSEngland/ AboutNHSservices/mental-health-services-explained/Pages/ accessing%20services.aspx.**

If you're keen to get help but reluctant to talk with your doctor, you might find it useful to access the **British Association for Counselling and Psychotherapy's** (BACP)

'Find a Therapist' directory. This lets you find qualified and professional counselling services in your local area.

Website: **www.bacp.co.uk/about-therapy/how-to-find-a-therapist/**

Samaritans is a registered charity based in the UK and Ireland. They provide confidential emotional support to anyone who is suicidal or despairing. Their confidential telephone helpline is available 24 hours a day, 7 days a week.

Helpline: **08457 90 90 90**
Email: **jo@samaritans.org**
Website: **www.samaritans.org**

Mind is a charity that provides advice and support to empower anyone who is experiencing a mental health problem. It campaigns to improve services, raise awareness and promote understanding of mental health.

Mind provides information on a range of topics including the types of mental health problems, and where to get help, as well as medication and alternative treatments.

Their contact lines are open from 9am to 6pm (Monday to Friday, expect for bank holidays).

Helpline: **0300 123 3393**
Text: **86463**
Email: **info@mind.org.uk**
Website: **www.mind.org.uk**

Mind also has a **Legal Line** for legal information and general advice on mental health related law covering mental health, mental capacity, community care, human rights and discrimination/equality related to mental health issues.

This line is open from 9am to 6pm
(Monday to Friday, expect bank holidays).
Telephone: **0300 466 6463**
Email: **Legal@mind.org.uk**
Website: **www.mind.org.uk**

The Men's Health Forum is an independent and authoritative voice for male health in England and Wales, tackling the issues and inequalities affecting the health and wellbeing of men and boys.

Telephone: **020 7922 7908**
Website: **www.menshealthforum.org.uk**

Mental Health First Aid is an organization whose mission is to train one in ten people in England in Mental Health First Aid (MHFA) skills.

This will empower people to care for themselves and others and help to reduce the stigma associated with mental health, breaking down barriers and enabling people to access the support they need to stay well, recover or manage their symptoms so they can thrive in learning, work and life.

Telephone: **020 7250 8062**
Email. **info@mhfaengland.org**
Website: **www.mhfaengland.org**

Citizens Advice provides free, independent, confidential and impartial advice to everyone on their rights and responsibilities. Their aim is to provide the advice people need for the problems they face and improve the policies and practices that affect people's lives.

Website: **www.citizensadvice.org.uk**

Stonewall is an organization that campaigns for the equality of lesbian, gay, bisexual and trans people across Britain. It provides information and support for LGBT communities and their allies on topics from coming out to information on your rights and how to take action against discrimination.

Website: **www.stonewall.org.uk**

TransUnite is a comprehensive resource for people in the UK searching for support in the transgender community. It offers a directory that can connect you with an established network of trans support groups.

Email. **info@transunite.co.uk**
Website: **www.transunite.co.uk**

Business in the Community (BITC) exists to build healthy communities with successful businesses at their heart. It is a business-led membership organization that is made up of progressive businesses of all sizes who understand that the prosperity of business and society are mutually dependent.

Workplace campaigns undertaken by BITC are committed to ensuring that age, gender, race and wellbeing do not limit an employee's engagement and success in the workplace and includes a focus on mental health in the workplace.

Telephone: **020 7566 8650**
Email: **information@bitc.org.uk**
Website: **wellbeing.bitc.org.uk**

Drinkaware is an independent charity working to reduce alcohol misuse and harm in the UK, helping people to make better choices about drinking.

Telephone: **020 7766 9900**
Email: **contact@drinkaware.co.uk**
Website: **www.drinkaware.co.uk**

GamCare is the UK's leading national provider of free information, advice and support for anyone affected by problem gambling.

Telephone: **0808 8020 133**
Email: **info@gamcare.org.uk**
Website: **www.gamcare.org.uk**

Gamblers Anonymous is an international organization devoted to helping people stop gambling. The organization's website is a gateway to a network of international meetings.

Website: **www.gamblersanonymous.org/ga/**

Student Minds is the UK's student mental health charity, empowering students and members of the university community to look after their own mental health, support others and create change.

Email: **info@studentminds.org.uk**
Website: **www.studentminds.org.uk**

There are also plenty of resources for organizations and employers to help improve the mental health and wellbeing of their people. The **UK Employee Assistance Professionals Association**, for example, is a not-for-profit organization that represents the interests of individuals and organizations concerned with employee assistance, psychological health and wellbeing.

Email: **info@eapa.org.uk**
Website: **www.eapa.org.uk**

Similarly, **COHPA** – the commercial occupational health providers' association – is an organization that provides information for employers seeking to access effective occupational health, as well as helping to make a link between employers and occupational health providers.

Email: **info@cohpa.co.uk**
Website: **cohpa.co.uk**

OUR FAVOURITE MENTAL HEALTH APPS

As well as the very many organizations and experts that are out there to help manage mental health, apps are a fantastic way to access support, latest information and research and practical help to nurture positive mental health.

Here is a run-down on some of our favourites – but bear in mind some of the advice we shared earlier on social media and carefully managing how much you rely on it!

These apps are available to download from the App Store or Google Play. Please refer to each app for subscription and in-app purchase information.

- **Calm** – one of the leading apps for meditating and mindfulness, offering access to guided meditations that can help manage anxiety, lower stress and sleep better.

Website: **www.calm.com**

- **Headspace** – access resources to live a healthier, happier and more rested life, helping subscribers to meditate and live mindfully through themed sessions on everything including stress, sleep and anxiety, as well as support for sudden meltdowns.

Website: **www.headspace.com**

- **Elefriends** – available from mental health charity Mind, this is a supportive online community that lets you be you, and offers a safe place to listen, share and be heard when you're struggling with your mental health.

Website: **www.elefriends.org.uk**

- **Catch It** – this NHS app is a great way to capture your mood and is designed to help manage feelings like anxiety and depression by teaching you to look at problems in a different way and turn negative thoughts into positive ones.

Website: **www.nhs.uk/apps-library**

OUR BENEFICIARIES

This book has been jointly funded and sponsored by Royal Mail Group and Optima Health. All proceeds from the sale of this book are being donated to the following two charities:

The Rowland Hill Fund
The Rowland Hill Fund was established in 1882 as a memorial to Sir Rowland Hill, the great postal reformer and founder of the modern British postal service, who retired as Secretary of the Post Office in 1864.

Over the years, the fund has helped thousands of individuals. In its early days, before the existence of the 'Welfare State' or the introduction of occupational pensions, organizations such as the fund were often the only place people could turn when in financial distress. However, although welfare provision is now an accepted part of society, there is still financial distress, and the Rowland Hill Fund is still a vibrant organization.

The fund deals with a wide range of cases and the diverse nature of the help it is able to provide reflects an ongoing need for the financial support it gives.

Due to the ever-increasing cost of living, the fund encounters many situations that produce genuine difficulty for individuals and their families. It is uniquely positioned to help Royal Mail, Post Office Limited and any of the associated companies' people who are in financial distress.

For more information, go to **www.rowlandhillfund.org**

Mind

Mind provides advice and support to empower anyone experiencing a mental health problem. They campaign to improve services, raise awareness and promote understanding. They won't give up until everyone experiencing a mental health problem gets support and respect.

For more information, go to **www.mind.org.uk**

ABOUT THE AUTHORS

Andrew and Shaun have previously co-authored *Positive Male Mind: Overcoming Mental Health Problems* which supports men and those that care about them by providing insight, advice and tips on what can be done at a very practical level to make men's mental health much more positive.

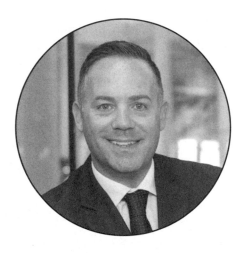

DR SHAUN DAVIS

Shaun is Global Director of Safety, Health, Wellbeing and Sustainability for Royal Mail Group.

He is also a Chartered Director and Fellow of the Institute of Directors, a Chartered Fellow of The Institution of Occupational Safety and Health, a Chartered Fellow of

The Chartered Institute of Personnel and Development and a Fellow of The International Institute of Risk and Safety Management. He was also appointed Honorary Assistant Professor at the University of Nottingham's School of Medicine in February 2018.

Shaun holds six master's degrees: an MA in Leadership & Culture Change, an MBA, an MA in Marketing & Innovation, an MSc in Workplace Health & Wellbeing, an MA in Strategic Human Resource Management and a Master of Laws (LLM).

Research for his doctorate in Coaching and Mentoring explored the relationship between coaching, wellbeing and organizational culture, examining how coaching influences employee wellbeing and productivity.

Shaun is currently a trustee of three charities: The Rowland Hill Fund (Trustee and Deputy Chair), The Men's Health Forum and The Society of Occupational Medicine. He is also a member of the Business in the Community (BITC) Workwell Leadership Team and a Member of the National Forum on Health and Wellbeing in the Workplace. In addition, he acts as Vice Chair and Director of Strategy for the pan-European mental health campaign 'Target Depression in the Workplace'.[46]

Follow Shaun on Twitter at **@DrShaunDavis**

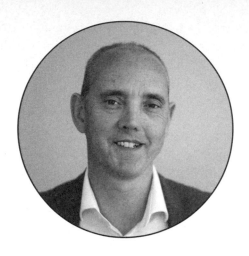

ANDREW KINDER

Andrew is a Chartered Counselling & Chartered Occupational Psychologist and Registered Coach with the British Psychological Society as well as the Past Chair of the British Association for Counselling and Psychotherapy's Workplace Division [www.bacpworkplace.org.uk]. He was awarded a Fellowship from BACP for his contributions to workplace counselling. He is an Associate Fellow of the British Psychological Society and a Registered Practitioner Psychologist with the Health and Care Professions Council. Andrew has two diplomas in counselling, an MSc in Occupational Psychology and is a Senior Accredited BACP Counsellor.

He has published two academic books with co-editors Professor Sir Cary Cooper and Rick Hughes – *Employee Wellbeing Support: A workplace Resource* and *International*

Handbook of Workplace Trauma Support. His latest works, again with the same co-editors, are the self-help books *The Crisis Book* and *The Wellbeing Workout*.

Andrew is an experienced practitioner with 25 years' experience. He works as a psychologist, counsellor, mediator and coach. He has been published widely and is particularly interested in the management of work-related mental health and trauma within organizations. He is currently the Professional Head of Mental Health Services at Optima Health. He has been instrumental in the introduction of early intervention programmes in a number of large organizations, relating to employee engagement, remote working, wellbeing strategies, psychological trauma and employee wellbeing.

He is currently Vice Chair of the UK Employee Assistance Professionals Association [www.eapa.org.uk] and in early 2018 the group awarded him an Emeritus Membership for his work in the employee assistance industry. Andrew is also a Trustee with the British Association for Counselling and Psychotherapy.

For more information on Optima Health,
go to **www.optimahealth.co.uk**

More information on Andrew can be found
at **www.andrewkinder.co.uk** or follow him on LinkedIn at **www.linkedin.com/in/andrew-kinder-31a75712**

ABOUT THE BOOK'S SPONSORS

ROYAL MAIL GROUP

Royal Mail is the UK's pre-eminent delivery company. We deliver more letters and parcels to more addresses in the UK, than all of our competitors combined.

We are proud to deliver a 'one price goes anywhere' service on a range of letters and parcels to around 30 million addresses, across the UK, six-days-a-week, in our role as the UK's sole designated Universal Service Provider. Royal Mail has deep cultural roots and these have helped to shape the history of the UK and the way the world communicates for over 500 years.

We also make a very significant contribution to the wider UK economy, Through UK Parcels, International & Letters (UKPIL), our impact and value-add, including through employment and procurement, is significant.

General Logistics Systems (GLS), our pan-European parcels business, operates one of the largest ground-based deferred parcel delivery networks in Europe.

For more information, go to **www.royalmailgroup.com**

OPTIMA HEALTH

Optima Health is a leading UK occupational health and wellbeing company. We help organizations and their people perform at their best by managing their health.

We have an extensive employee team of over 450 occupational health practitioners in the UK: consultant physicians, occupational health nurses, occupational therapists, physiotherapists, counsellors, psychologists, technicians, registered nurses and physiologists.

We work across a range of sectors, both public and private. Within the private sector we specialise in the energy and utilities, construction, manufacturing, rail, transport and financial sectors. We also provide services to organizations providing emergency services and are one of the largest providers to the NHS, as well as to central and local government in occupational health and Employee Assistance Programmes.

We know that one size doesn't fit all. So, our preference is to work with organizations to understand their requirements. This way we can create integrated, compelling and multidisciplinary solutions where, together, we focus on outcomes, measuring value and return on investment for the organization.

For more information, go to **www.optimahealth.co.uk**

REFERENCES

1. C. Deverill and M. King (2009), 'Common mental disorders', in Adult Psychiatric Morbidity Survey.

2. https://time-to-change.org.uk

3. https://wellbeing.bitc.org.uk/all-resources/toolkits/sleep-and-recovery-toolkit

4. https://www.gov.uk/government/publications/the-public-health-burden-of-alcohol-evidence-review

5. https://www.ons.gov.uk/peoplepopulationandcommunity/healthandsocialcare/drugusealcoholandsmoking/datasets/adultdrinkinghabits

6. https://www.drinkaware.co.uk/alcohol-facts/health-effects-of-alcohol/mental-health/alcohol-and-mental-health/

7. http://stepup-international.co.uk/can-drinking-be-classed-as-self-harm/

8. https://digital.nhs.uk/data-and-information/publications/statistical/health-survey-for-england/health-survey-for-england-2016

9. Holt-Lunstadt, J., Smith, T.B. & Layton, J.B. (2010). Social Relationships and Mortality Risk: a meta-analytic review. PLoS Medicine 7 (7): e1000316. doi:10.1371/journal.pmed.1000316

10. https://mashable.com/2017/08/07/3-billion-global-social-media-users/?europe=true#o0uBlW9Cuaqf

11. https://journals.sagepub.com/doi/full/10.1177/2167702617723376

12. https://www.huffingtonpost.co.uk/2014/07/25/social-media-mental-healt_n_5619728. html?ir=UK+Tech&guccounter=1&guce_referrer=aHR0cDovL3d3dy5iYmMuY29tL2Z1d HVyZS9zdG9yeS8yMDE4MDEwNC1pcy1zb2NpYWwtbWVkaWEtYmFkLWZvci15b3Ud GhlLWV2aWRlbmNlLWFuZC10aGUtdW5rbm93bnM&guce_referrer_sig=AQAAALp2db 3PJOgmbWHYq6gSqMP6gCfbREqHflfsguXxiMAD-j5pdxnY9O1FdFt69jrpK9QuZq66Ve UQL3p1SEvZy8yLFVCdk13uvfGRNW0SCj5H1oTZofAjNYP073nR-WW1kmmT5rYl9u G9C3FeK2MNqNhuFCEVE7g4JKhVS2X4bO9

13. https://www.theweek.co.uk/93630/body-clock-disruption-linked-to-depression

14. https://www.ajpmonline.org/article/S0749-3797(17)30016-8/fulltext

15. https://munews.missouri.edu/news-releases/2015/0203-if-facebook-use-causes-envy-depression-could-follow/

16. https://www.walesonline.co.uk/news/wales-news/swansea-professor-says-social-media-13121701

17. https://www.rcpsych.ac.uk/mental-health/problems-disorders/debt-and-mental-health

18. http://www.moneyandmentalhealth.org/wp-content/uploads/2017/05/MMHPIOverstretched-Overdrawn-Underserved.pdf

19. https://www.rcpsych.ac.uk/mental-health/problems-disorders/problem-gambling

20. https://www.theguardian.com/society/2019/mar/13/problem-gamblers-at-15-times-higher-risk-of-suicide-study-finds

21. https://www.gamcare.org.uk/

22. http://www.gamblersanonymous.org/ga/content/about-us

23. https://assets.publishing.service.gov.uk/government/uploads/system/uploads/attachment_data/file/539682/160719_REPORT_LGBT_evidence_review_NIESR_FINALPDF.pdf

24. Zietsch, B.P., Verweij, K.J.H., Heath, A.C., Madden, P.A.F., Martin, N.G., Nelson, E.C., & Lynskey, M.T. (2012). Do shared etiological factors contribute to the relationship between sexual orientation and depression? *Psychological Medicine*, 42(3), 521–532.

25. Liu, R., & Mustanski, B. (2012). Suicidal Ideation and Self-Harm in Lesbian, Gay, Bisexual, and Transgender Youth. *American Journal of Preventative Medicine*, 42(3), 221–228

26. Marshal, M.P., Friedman, M.S., Stall, R., & Thompson, A.L. (2009). Individual trajectories of substance use in lesbian, gay and bisexual youth and heterosexual youth. *Addiction*, 104, 974–981

27. https://www.mind.org.uk/media/5204367/mind-lgbtqplusguide-2016webres.pdf

28. https://wellbeing.bitc.org.uk/all-resources/research-articles/working-pride-report-issues-affecting-lgbt-people-workplace

29. https://www.rethink.org/living-with-mental-illness/wellbeing-physical-health/lgbtplus-mental-health/issues

30. https://www.rethink.org/advice-information/living-with-mental-illness/wellbeing-physical-health/lgbtplus-mental-health/

31. https://www.pinknews.co.uk/2016/12/11/study-finds-40-of-transgender-people-have-attempted-suicide/

32. www.hse.gov.uk

33. Rick J, O'Regan S, Kinder A (November 2006) *Early Intervention following trauma – a controlled longitudinal study at Royal Mail Group*, Institute of Employment Studies, Report 435.

34. https://www.nice.org.uk/guidance/ng116

35. https://www.ons.gov.uk/peoplepopulationandcommunity/wellbeing/bulletins/personalandeconomicwellbeingintheuk/april2019#dashboard-of-well-being-indicators

36. McManus S, Bebbington P, Jenkins R, Brugha T. (eds.) (2016) Mental health and wellbeing in England: Adult Psychiatric Morbidity Survey 2014. Leeds: NHS Digital, see http://digital.nhs.uk/catalogue/PUB21748]

37. https://www.samaritans.org/news/suicide-kills-three-times-more-people-road-traffic-accidents-we-urgently-need-act

38. https://wellbeing.bitc.org.uk/sites/default/files/business_in_the_community_suicide_prevention_toolkit_0.pdf

39. https://yougov.co.uk/topics/lifestyle/articles-reports/2016/08/09/quarter-britains-students-are-afflicted-mental-hea

40. https://www.telegraph.co.uk/news/2018/04/12/universities-have-suicide-problem-students-taking-lives-overtakes/

41. https://www.apa.org/monitor/apr03/pluses

42. https://www.nhs.uk/conditions/menopause/

43. https://assets.publishing.service.gov.uk/government/uploads/system/uploads/attachment_data/file/209510/hwwb-is-work-good-for-you-exec-summ.pdf

44. https://www.mentalhealth.org.uk/news/38-brits-fear-revealing-mental-health-problem-work-would-jeopardise-their-career

45. https://sleepfoundation.org/sleep-tools-tips/healthy-sleep-tips

46. www.targetdepression.com

ABOUT THE BOOK

Improve, nurture and protect your mental health at home, in life and in the workplace.

We all face challenges in our lives when it comes to mental health, regardless of age, sexual or gender orientation and too often we can be guilty of taking our mental health for granted. This book will help you to take charge of your mental health, improving your understanding of some of the most common mental health conditions and explain how to manage your mental health at work and through challenging life milestones.

When it comes to mental health, stress, work/life balance, resilience and managing change, Dr Shaun Davis and Andrew Kinder are leading practitioners who have more than 50 years' experience between them.

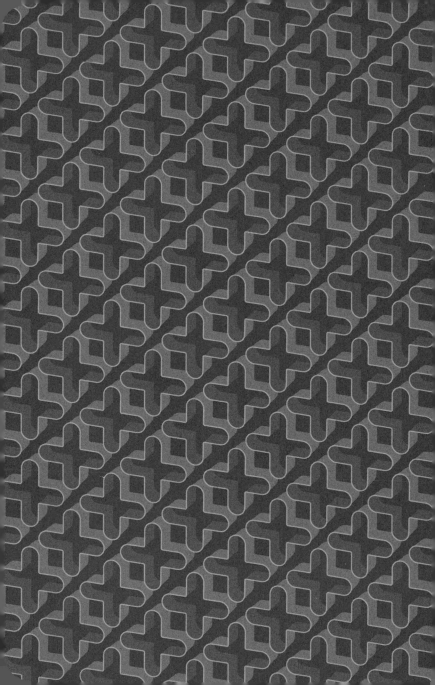